What People Are Saying About
The Schwarzbein Principle . . .

"Dr. Schwarzbein i   in the vanguard of new   icine. Her approach to staving off the accelerated aging process works. Anyone who has battled weight problems, heart disease, osteoporosis, diabetes or high cholesterol levels will benefit from this incredible book."

Suzanne Somers
actress, entertainer, author

"When I had my liver transplant four years ago, I was diagnosed as diabetic and knew I had to make some serious eating and lifestyle changes. To my relief, after reading *The Schwarzbein Principle*, I found that those changes were going to be fairly easy. I could eat all of the red meat, eggs, butter and cream I wanted. I lost twenty-five pounds in five months, and today I look and feel better. My cholesterol level is the best it has ever been and I'm healthier than I have been in years. I no longer need to inject insulin and my diabetes is under control."

Larry Hagman
actor, director, producer

"A long-overdue guide to healthy eating based on scientific principles. Dr. Schwarzbein has taken fundamental physiology and made it literally digestible for the general public."

Eric McFarland, Ph.D., M.D.
University of California, Santa Barbara

THE SCHWARZBEIN PRINCIPLE

The Truth About
LOSING WEIGHT, BEING HEALTHY AND FEELING YOUNGER

Diana Schwarzbein, M.D.,
Nancy Deville

Health Communications, Inc.
Deerfield Beach, Florida

www.hci-online.com

Library of Congress Cataloging-in-Publication Data

Schwarzbein, Diana
    The Schwarzbein principle: the truth about losing weight, being healthy and feeling younger / Diana Schwarzbein and Nancy Deville.
      p.   cm.
    ISBN 1-55874-680-3 (trade paper)
    1. Sugar-free diet.   2. Nutrition.   3. Health.   4. Weight loss.
I. Deville, Nancy.   II. Title
RM237.85.S35   1999
613—dc21   99-24102
                                                  CIP

©1999 by Diana Schwarzbein and Nancy Deville

ISBN 1-55874-680-3

Publisher: Health Communications, Inc.
              3201 S.W. 15th Street
              Deerfield Beach, FL 33442-8190

Original sketches for illustrations by Wynn Kapit, Diana Schwarzbein, M.D., and Nancy Deville
Illustrations by Orien Armstrong and Larissa Hise
Cover design by Lisa Camp
Author photos by Alice Williams

For Larry,
Mami and Papi,
Viviana, Sergio, Gabriella,
Audrey, Dick, Danielle, Jacob,
Alexis, Keith and Rachel

—DIANA SCHWARZBEIN, M.D.

For John

—NANCY DEVILLE

Contents

Acknowledgments xi

Introduction xv

PART I: AGING

One: What Is the Accelerated Metabolic Aging Process? 3

Two: Human Survival Depends on Hormones and Fat 17

Three: Humans Are Part of the Food Chain 29

Four: The Low-Serotonin State:
   The Common Denominator 39

PART II: CHOLESTEROL AND FAT

Five: Dietary Cholesterol and Fat Are Essential to Life 61

Six: Why You Must Eat Cholesterol 67

PART III: HEART DISEASE, TYPE II DIABETES AND CANCER

Seven: Your Cholesterol Count Is Not the Final Word 75

Eight: What About the Good HDLs? 85

Nine: The *Real* Risk Factors for a Heart Attack 93

Ten: Two Packs of Cigarettes a Day x Fifty Years =
  Accelerated Metabolic Aging 103

Eleven: Cancer and the High-Insulin Lifestyle 109

PART IV: ACHIEVING A BALANCED DIET

Twelve: Carbohydrates Are Sugar 119

Thirteen: Fat Does Not Make You Fat 127

Fourteen: Gaining Body Fat on a Low-Fat Diet 133

Fifteen: Dispelling Low-Fat Beliefs 141

PART V: EATING DISORDERS

Sixteen: Diet Scams 149

Seventeen: Dr. Schwarzbein, Sugar Junkie 163

Eighteen: You *Can* Be Too Thin 173

Nineteen: Overfed and Undernourished 189

Twenty: Children Do Not Have to Be Overweight 195

PART VI: THE VEGETARIAN DIET

Twenty-One: The Committed Vegetarian 203

Twenty-Two: The Body Is Interconnected 209

PART VII: CHANGING YOUR LIFESTYLE

Twenty-Three: Changing Her Lifestyle Without Suffering 217

PART VIII: THE HEALING AND MAINTENANCE PROGRAMS

Twenty-Four: The Schwarzbein Nutrition and
  Lifestyle Programs 223

Twenty-Five: The Schwarzbein Healing and
  Maintenance Nutritional Programs 241

Twenty-Six: What Not to Eat 277

Twenty-Seven: Planning Your Meals 289

References 339

Index 353

About the Authors 365

Illustrations

1-1   How Insulin Resistance Develops 9

3-1   The Food Chain 32

3-2   The USDA Food Pyramid 34

3-3   The Schwarzbein Square 35

6-1   Following Carbohydrates Through Your System 68

9-1   The Solid, Continuous Wall of Plaque 96

9-2   The Liquid Core of Cholesterol Plaque 97

12-1   How Glucagon Works 120

12-2   How Insulin Works 121

27-1   What Your Groceries Used to Look Like 290

27-2   What Your Groceries Look Like on the
       Schwarzbein Program 291

27-3   What a Vegetarian's Groceries Look Like on the
       Schwarzbein Program 307

Acknowledgments

This book was made possible by the support, hard work and encouragement of many.

Dr. Schwarzbein owes a debt of gratitude to John Nicoloff, M.D., for teaching her to be an independent thinker. We both thank all of Dr. Schwarzbein's patients who participated in her initial and ongoing clinical trials. A special thanks to Horacio Hojman, M.D., for his assistance in gathering medical literature.

Nancy Deville wishes to thank Cathy Quinn, Ph.D., for her wisdom and affection, without which the writing of this book would not have been possible.

Our deepest appreciation goes to the people who shared with us in detail their own healing experiences. This book would not have been the same without their contributions.

We are grateful to John Davis, D.B.A., for painstakingly editing our many manuscripts and for his extensive and insightful comments that helped us make the text clear. We appreciate the many times we relied on his resources at the Owner Managed Business Institute (OMBI) offices to run off copies of the manuscript, send faxes, use the Pitney Bowes and the numerous and sundry office supplies that trickled our way over the months. Joy Morrison and Reneé Perez at OMBI were consistently cheerful and helpful in those many "small things" that tended to pile up.

Our artist Orien Armstrong realized our vision of a clear, compelling and accessible book. Harold "Wardie" Ward worked computer magic on the finished drawings as changes became necessary. We also thank Wynn Kapit for his original sketches of many of the illustrations.

David Stanley, our computer technician, responded to all our needs with an "above and beyond the call of duty" attitude, not to mention a great sense of humor.

Robin Marzi, R.D., Sheridan Eldridge and Adele Staal all gave tremendous focus and attention to analyzing and organizing our mass of information. Sheridan's organizational and cooking skills made it possible for us to get out a first draft in record time.

Thanks to our attorneys Gideon Cashman and Bob Stein for their generosity and expertise.

Our thanks would not be complete without acknowledging the many people who read and commented on drafts of the manuscript as it evolved: Edison Schwarzbein, Ph.D.; Martha Schwarzbein, M.A.; Nadine Saubers, R.N.; Louise Moore; Nancy and Dick Graham; Sheila and Nick Fowler; Audrey Schwarzbein, M.D.; Dick Graham, M.D.; Marsha Wayne; Glenn Miller, M.D.; Marjorie Gies, M.D.; and Shireen Fatemi, M.D.

Many thanks to the staff at the Endocrinology Institute, both past and present: Olga Barraza; Tammy Bateson; Helen Curhan, M.P.H., R.D.; Amy Decker; Debbie Hensler, L.V.N.; Jennifer Hoyt, P.A.; Kathi Newall, R.D.; Allison Mayer-Oakes, M.D.; Cindy Ordway; Leilani Price, R.D.; Sue Reardon, R.N.; Keith Sersland; Andrew Shapiro; Susanne Shelledy; Kelli Tatlock; Doris Vargas; Jane Westerman; Martha Wilkens, R.D., Patti Williams, R.N., and Janice Zagarra, R.N.

We are indebted to Pat Frederick for her unflagging enthusiasm for our project. Her grasp of the English language and expertise at copy editing inspired our confidence as she put our manuscript through a thorough final edit. We also thank Grace Rachow and Fran Davis for thoughtful editorial input and support along the way. Thanks to Micki Taylor for an exceptional job on the index and Jill Kern, Ph.D., for her work on the References.

Thanks to Virginia Loy for her support, and to John Bury for doing a fine job of administration.

Our unique publishing story, a long and winding tale, took a promising twist with an introduction to Jack Canfield by Russell Bishop who, needless to say, we are deeply indebted to. In turn, we must thank Jack Canfield for his role in getting our manuscripts to Peter Vegso at Health Communications, Inc. It is nearly impossible to express our gratitude and appreciation to our agent, Barbara Neighbors Deal, who has done so much for us, including handling the many details that went into making our publishing deal. Not only has she served us well as an agent and friend, but her results on the program made all of our hard work seem worthwhile.

In the end, however, our books would not have been published if not for Peter Vegso. We thank Peter for believing in our project, and for his infectious enthusiasm.

We are also grateful to Peter's staff: Christine Belleris, editorial co-director; Allison Janse, associate editor; Kim Weiss and Maria Konicki in PR; Lisa Camp for the cover design; Erica Orloff, Bob Land and Mary Ellen Hettinger for their editing and proofreading expertise; Lawna Oldfield for the book's text design; Robert Solomon, attorney; and Theresa Peluso, executive assistant, for all of their expertise, support and hard work in getting the book to press.

We also thank Lisa Ekus and Merrilyn Lewis at Lisa Ekus Public Relations for their wonderful efforts on our behalf.

And not to be forgotten, "*The Schwarzbein Principle* Chef" Evelyn Jacob Jaffe, for coming through when we needed her.

Most of all we thank our husbands, Larry Mousouris and John Davis, for their love, understanding and patience, for putting up with our impossible hours, and for their unflagging encouragement and enthusiasm for this project.

Introduction

Researching the Schwarzbein Principle

In medical training, I was taught that a low-fat diet high in complex carbohydrates prevented weight gain and disease. I believed what my professors said. Early on, I advocated low-fat diets. But this soon changed. I now teach my patients to balance their meals. Let me tell you how this all came about.

In July 1990, I had just finished nine years of medical training at the University of Southern California. My training was in endocrinology and metabolism, and I was ready to go out and help the world.

I accepted a position at a prestigious medical clinic in Santa Barbara, California. The clinic was famous for having been the premier diabetes center in the United States during the 1920s.

I was excited about starting my new position, but I was not thrilled that all my new patients would be Type II diabetics.[1] My area of expertise was "esoteric" endocrine diseases—hypothyroidism, adrenal and pituitary problems—conditions where the patient's symptoms could be reversed.

Type II diabetics did not get better. I had seen too many diabetics

---

[1] *This story begins with my work with Type II diabetes. You may believe that Type II diabetes does not pertain to you. But it does. Please read on.*

have legs amputated, too many who required kidney dialysis or who had scars down the middle of their chests from coronary bypass grafting. Working with diabetics meant that I would have to watch people inevitably get sicker and die. But having accepted the challenge, I committed myself to giving patients my best care.

Because the patients were all new to me, I spent a full hour with each one, obtaining a detailed history. I will never forget the anxiety I felt when they would begin by saying, "I hope you won't tell me the same thing all the other doctors have said. It just doesn't work for me." They complained of higher blood-sugar levels and high blood pressure, despite medication, and of chronic fatigue, weight gain and abnormal cholesterol profiles.

I heard many stories of patients going for yearly physical exams and being diagnosed with diabetes incidentally. Chemistry panels had come back with a red flag of high blood sugar—diabetes. These newly diagnosed diabetics were put on the American Diabetes Association (ADA) diet—a low-calorie, high-carbohydrate, low-fat, low-protein program. The diet stressed fruit, milk, bread and very little fat. It was very complicated. They had to measure everything they ate—proteins and fats, as well as carbohydrates. These patients had stuck to this diet, only to see their conditions worsen.

Diabetes was considered genetic. The fact that these patients had gotten worse was considered part of the progressive genetic nature of the disease. It was thought that once a person developed diabetes, it could not be reversed. Part of the "standard of care" was to keep diabetics' blood sugar under control to enable them to live relatively normal lives.

Physicians manipulated insulin doses to bring patients' blood sugars down. But my patients complained, "When my other doctors gave me insulin, I gained weight." That made sense because insulin is a fat-storing hormone. The patients' weight gain along with high insulin levels had caused increased blood pressure. Many had been prescribed drugs to lower blood pressure, which in some cases made their blood sugars worse. It was a vicious cycle. They injected insulin, but their blood-sugar levels did not improve. They gained weight and required more insulin. And their cholesterol levels were getting worse. Here were patients who had been accidentally diagnosed with diabetes when they felt relatively well, and now, after following the "standard of diabetes care," they felt terrible.

After listening to their stories I thought, *My God, we are making diabetics worse!*

I remember the sinking feeling as I told them, "I understand why you're upset about what has happened to you. But I would have asked you to follow the exact same regimen the other doctors have been prescribing. At this moment, I don't know what else to tell you, but I'm going to help you get better any way I can."

I decided for the time being to get a baseline. "You're going to monitor your blood sugar seven times a day at home with a blood-sugar monitoring device," I instructed. "Before you eat, an hour after you eat and at bedtime. Write everything down. Everything you're feeling, everything you eat, activities, blood-sugar levels and any other observations. I'll see you again in a week."

When they returned after monitoring their habits, my patients all told me, "It's the food I'm eating!"

It was clear. These patients were monitoring their blood sugar. When they did a "finger blood-sugar stick" in the morning, their blood sugar was normal. Then they ate a perfect ADA breakfast—a bowl of shredded wheat with non-fat milk, a banana and a glass of orange juice—and watched their blood sugar rise one hundred to two hundred points. (A normal blood-sugar response to any meal is no more than ten to twenty points.)

Something they were eating was causing the problem. It could not be the protein. Protein will eventually turn into sugar, but not that quickly. It could not be the fat—they were eating hardly any fat—and fats do not turn into sugar that quickly either. Carbohydrates are the only nutrient group that can be converted into sugar so fast. All carbohydrates are recognized as sugar by the body, whether they are in the form of grains, starches, dairy, fruits or sweets. I suddenly recognized that by recommending a high-carbohydrate diet, *we were giving sugar to diabetics.*

In order to understand why sugar is so destructive to diabetics you need to appreciate the central role of insulin in human physiology. Insulin is the hormone responsible for tightly regulating the amount of sugar going to the brain after you eat. Insulin accomplishes this in two ways: First, the presence of insulin alerts the liver to incoming high amounts of sugar so that the liver does not let this high sugar pass through to the brain. Second, insulin stows away sugar into cells, thereby decreasing blood-sugar levels. Also, when sugar is stowed, insulin levels normalize. This system keeps blood sugars and insulin levels balanced.

But Type II diabetics are "insulin resistant," which means that the cells will not allow insulin to unload sugar from the bloodstream. Because the cells do not respond to insulin, the pancreas reacts by secreting even more insulin in an attempt to open up the closed cells. This results in Type II diabetics having both high insulin levels and high blood-sugar levels. If you then ask diabetics to eat more carbohydrates (as in the ADA diet), it further increases both their blood-sugar levels and insulin levels.

Requiring diabetics with high blood-sugar levels to follow a high-sugar diet did not make sense. But how could I challenge the ADA? I reasoned that the ADA diet must have been thoroughly researched— they could not be recommending diets that were making people sicker! But all of my Type II diabetic patients returned with the same observations: The ADA diet was causing their blood sugars to rise to dangerous levels.

I decided to see what would happen to my patients' blood-sugar levels if I put them on a "zero"-carbohydrate diet. I asked them to eliminate all obvious carbohydrate foods, such as potatoes, rice, legumes, cereals, breads, fruit, low-fat yogurt, milk and, of course, refined sugar.

Since foods are often a combination of fats, proteins and carbohydrates, if a food caused a rise in their blood sugars we classified it in the carbohydrate category. For example, most people think that milk is all protein, when in fact the amount of carbohydrates in four ounces of milk drives a diabetic's blood sugar up approximately one hundred points. With this method, the main ingredient of a food and whether it raised blood-sugar levels dictated whether it should be considered a protein, a fat, a nonstarchy vegetable or a carbohydrate.

Because I did not want my patients to go hungry, I added some protein and fats back to their diet. At the time, I still thought that a low-fat diet was healthier, so I asked them to use low-fat dairy products, and to eat egg substitutes, mostly fish and chicken and small amounts of red meat.

I also educated my patients about insulin levels. Eliminating obvious carbohydrates for one week would rapidly lower their insulin levels, and they would have to reduce their diabetes medicines accordingly to avoid low blood-sugar reactions.

One week later, the first group of patients returned for an evaluation. I looked at the blood sugar numbers they had recorded. Their progress was astounding. I said, "This is unbelievable!"

Some confessed, "Dr. Schwarzbein, I've been cheating. I love red meat and when you said I could have some, I ate it every night for a week."

The "cheaters" were eating real mayonnaise, real cheese, real eggs and steak every day—foods that had been forbidden for so long they could not resist them. Their blood-sugar numbers had fallen dramatically. In fact, the biggest improvements were seen in the patients who "cheated" the most.

By cutting carbohydrates from their diets and adding proteins and fats, most patients (after an initial body-water loss) started losing one to two pounds of body fat per week. They ate fats and lost body fat. All came back to me and said, "I don't understand. I got fatter when I didn't eat fat. Now I'm eating fat and I'm losing weight."

Prior to this, these patients had high blood sugars, abnormal cholesterol panels, high blood pressure, weight gain, fatigue and constant hunger. As they followed the new dietary program their blood sugars normalized, so they were able to get off insulin and/or oral hypoglycemic agents (which treat high blood sugar). Their cholesterol levels improved, so I stopped their cholesterol-lowering medication. Their blood pressures came down, so I stopped their blood pressure medication. I was able to eliminate most of their drugs. They lost body fat and gained muscle mass. Their energy improved. They were not going hungry anymore. They felt great.

My diabetic patients were so happy with the improvements in their health that they began to refer family members to me. Although these referred patients were not diabetic, they suffered from fatigue, excessive body fat with decreased muscle mass, cholesterol problems, high blood pressure and even heart disease. I treated them with the same program. Body fat decreased and muscle mass increased, cholesterol levels normalized and blood pressures came down. They, too, felt great.

Word of my successful "diet" spread. I started treating patients who had the same symptoms as the first two groups but no family history of diabetes. These patients all related histories of poor diets and chronic dieting, including low-fat dieting. The program worked for them as well.

I began to see people with isolated conditions: bad cholesterol profiles, high blood-pressure problems or excessive body fat. I put them on the program, altered by then to include more oils, real eggs, real butter. I was amazed that the same program I used for my diabetics worked for all these people. Regardless of the patient's problem or illness, a balanced diet produced the same results—better health and decreased body fat.

I felt I needed to gain a better understanding of these relationships.

As I examined eating habits more closely I realized that, to reduce fat consumption as much as possible, many people cut down on proteins and ate more carbohydrates. Furthermore, since people had heard that complex carbohydrates are healthy and should form the bulk of their diets, they consumed *even more* carbohydrates.

Both medicine and the media had promoted the belief that eating a low-fat diet while increasing complex carbohydrates caused people to lose body fat and stay healthy. But I had yet to meet anyone who was healthy or thriving on a low-fat diet. Were the people who did well on low-fat diets so healthy that they had no need for doctors?

I searched the medical literature, looking for studies showing that low-fat diets are healthy. I was surprised to learn that there are no long-term studies showing such results. *But numerous studies concluded that fat is necessary to maintain good health.* And there are studies spanning three decades relating high insulin levels and heart disease, high insulin levels and hypertension, high insulin levels and excessive body-fat gain and other problems.

The light bulb turned on.

I was taught that diabetic patients have a very high rate of heart disease. Correspondingly, I had observed that diabetic patients frequently had a large scar down the middle of their chests. Frequently I found that these patients had heart bypass surgery *before* they were diagnosed with diabetes. The implications suddenly occurred to me! After a heart attack, people are told to go on a low-fat, high-carbohydrate diet—which increases both their blood-sugar and insulin levels. *The increases in blood sugar and insulin were turning heart patients into diabetics.* The newly created diabetics are then told to continue eating a diet high in carbohydrates, which further elevates their blood-sugar and insulin levels.

Next, we say to those diabetics, "Your blood sugar is too high, so you need to take insulin to bring that blood-sugar level down." But insulin injections produce even higher insulin levels—as well as increases in weight, blood pressure and the need for more insulin.

Furthermore, the studies I read substantiated a connection between prolonged high insulin levels and the degenerative diseases of aging, such as osteoarthritis, different types of cancer, cholesterol abnormalities, coronary artery disease, less lean body mass with excess body fat, high blood pressure, osteoporosis, stroke and Type II diabetes.

For example, it is known that insulin directs all the biochemical processes that lead to plaque formation in arteries; therefore, I recognized that prolonged high insulin levels lead to heart disease. It is also well known that prolonged high insulin levels could lead to insulin resistance; therefore, I also recognized that prolonged high insulin levels could also lead to Type II diabetes. These studies corroborated my clinical experience showing that elevated insulin is linked to disease. Unfortunately, medical studies had not pinpointed the causes of prolonged high insulin levels that led to insulin resistance. The connection between elevated insulin levels, heart disease and diabetes was assumed to be genetic. But I looked at it from a different angle. Since insulin resistance is connected to degenerative diseases, and since insulin resistance occurs naturally in the aging process, degenerative diseases of aging have to be linked to the aging process.

Because the degenerative diseases of aging were occurring in younger and younger individuals, I began to consider the possibility that degenerative diseases of aging were not genetic but *acquired.* By "acquired" I mean that people were accelerating their aging process through poor eating and lifestyle habits that raised insulin levels.

Furthermore, medical science had gotten stuck on the assumption that only some people have the high-insulin gene. Again we differed. My clinical experience demonstrated that people *acquired* (not inherited) insulin resistance—and that too many people were suffering from this condition. I became convinced that the *degenerative diseases of aging (which are the end result of insulin resistance) are accelerated by poor eating and lifestyle habits.* In other words, a genetic predisposition to disease is not a "guarantee" that you will develop that disease. Instead, what you do and how you live your life determines your risk for developing insulin resistance and the degenerative diseases of aging.

Of course there are genetic variables. For example, everyone (except Type I diabetics) secretes a different amount of insulin in response to various factors. However, this is clinically significant only when eating and lifestyle habits consistently cause insulin levels to rise. In other words, in a perfect world where everyone ate a balanced diet of real foods and avoided stimulants and stress, there would be no appreciable difference between those people who secreted more insulin and those who did not.

But this is not a perfect world. Poor eating and lifestyle habits have led to an imbalance of insulin levels; because the systems of the human body are interconnected, one imbalance creates another imbalance. This is beautifully illustrated by the current low-fat movement. Low-fat dieting upsets the balance within the human body by initially increasing insulin levels, in turn causing a cascade of hormone imbalances. The low-fat, high-carbohydrate movement promised long, healthy lives and trim, athletic bodies. But instead it caused prolonged high insulin levels, which in turn increased the number of people with heart disease, Type II diabetes, excessive weight gain and many more chronic conditions and diseases.

Here are the facts:

Claim: Eating fat makes you fat. If you do not eat fat, you cannot gain fat.

Fact: A low-fat diet makes you fat. Eating fat causes you to lose body fat and reach your ideal body composition. Furthermore, eating dietary fat is essential for life. Eating fat is essential for reproduction, for the regeneration of healthy tissues and for maintaining ideal body composition.

Claim: Eating fat and cholesterol adversely affects your cholesterol profile and puts you at risk for heart attacks.

Fact: Eating a low-fat diet causes heart attacks. High insulin levels produced by a low-fat, high-carbohydrate diet result in plaqueing of the arteries, because insulin directs all the biochemical processes that lead to plaque formation in arteries. Eating fat and cholesterol can prevent heart attacks by lowering insulin levels and switching off the internal production of cholesterol.

Claim: Eating fat causes cancer. Low-fat diets prevent cancer.

Fact: Low-fat diets (high in carbohydrates) cause insulin levels to rise too high—a growth factor and a major player in cancer-cell replication. Dietary fat lowers insulin levels. Dietary fat is also essential for hormone production, which in turn is essential for a healthy immune system. In other words, dietary fat provides the immune system with key components that fight the growth of cancer cells.

Claim: Eating fat increases your risk of high blood pressure (hypertension).

Fact: Cutting fat from your diet *increases* the risk of high blood pressure because, without fat, insulin levels rise higher in response to food. Insulin stimulates various biochemical processes that can lead to increased blood pressure.

Claim: A low-fat, high-carbohydrate diet, which is the current "standard of care" treatment for diabetes, makes patients healthier.

Fact: Long-term low-fat, high-carbohydrate dieting leads to insulin resistance and, if continued, results in Type II diabetes. This same diet makes diabetics sicker.

It is important to note that these claims are not backed up by long-term scientific studies. But the *facts* are supported by physiology and biochemistry (true science).

By focusing on physiology and biochemistry, and the evidence of my own clinical experience, I learned how prolonged high insulin levels set off a multitude of chain reactions that disrupt all other hormones and biochemical reactions at the cellular level. I termed this chronic disruption "accelerated metabolic aging," and recognized that it led to body-fat gain, chronic conditions and degenerative diseases.

Throughout the six-year period I have referred to above, I learned that there are other factors that raise insulin levels, both directly and indirectly, and that prolonged high insulin levels are caused not only by eating a low-fat, high-carbohydrate diet but also by stress, dieting, caffeine, alcohol, aspartame (an artificial sweetener), tobacco, steroids, stimulant and other recreational drugs, lack of exercise, excessive and/or unnecessary thyroid replacement therapy, and all over-the-counter and prescription drugs. These factors have become central in the eating and lifestyle habits that have prevailed over the last twenty years and that parallel the rise in the incidence of disease during this same period of time.

My program gradually expanded to include balanced nutrition, stress management, exercise, the elimination of stimulants and other drugs, and hormone replacement therapy—a complete program designed to balance insulin and all other hormone levels.

The Schwarzbein Principle was written to share this program with you—to tell the truth about losing weight, being healthy and feeling younger, by first focusing on this principle: *Degenerative diseases are not genetic but acquired. Because the systems of the human body are interconnected and because one imbalance creates another imbalance, poor eating and lifestyle habits, not genetics, are the cause of degenerative disease.*

I have seen what high-insulin eating and lifestyle habits do to people. People are getting fatter, sicker and more depressed. Indeed, it has not taken long—only two decades—to realize the repercussions of eliminating fat, one of the most important nutrient groups, from our diet and replacing real food with invented substances, processed foods and stimulants.

Moreover, American society's preoccupation with numbers—whether referring to chronological age, total cholesterol numbers or the number on the bathroom scale—has wrought devastating results. Many popular books offer programs that require time-consuming computations and obsessive measuring and focus on food. *But my experience with patients demonstrates that, ironically, the more a person obsesses about numbers the more likely he or she is to engage in harmful behaviors that generate chronic health problems and disease.* One of my goals as a physician is to change our culture's fixation on meaningless numbers to an emphasis on quality of life.

When people are told that poor health is genetic, they are more likely to tolerate illness and decreased quality of life as their lot. Along with this resignation comes increased body fat, depression and lethargy. Teaching people that health and vitality are within their grasp, and showing them how to achieve optimum health, is the key to the success of my program. When people understand that they have control over their health, they are motivated to make significant changes in habits.

As a physician, I hope to influence the medical profession so that more emphasis is placed on preventive medicine. Giving people the power to attain balance, to heal themselves and to avoid illness instills motivation, in addition to dramatically improving doctor-patient relationships and potentially revolutionizing the "standard of care."

This book could have been written around the many important studies that are cited in the References section. But the problem is that there is never going to be a perfect study. Questions always remain unanswered, no matter how many references you cite. And there are so many opposing theories that it would be virtually impossible to counter every one of them. I realize that I would have never come to my own conclusions about accelerated metabolic aging if I had focused on studies rather than true science. So I chose to write a book explaining how the body works at the cellular level, not a book based on other researchers' conclusions.

The truth is, anyone can prevent accelerated aging and disease, achieve ideal body composition and extend longevity. As you learn more about physiology and read the case histories that demonstrate my clinical experience (which shows that aging and disease are one and the same) you will understand how you can gain control over your health. My hope is that the information in this book will lead you to balanced nutrition and to a lifestyle that will regenerate and heal your body so as to prevent accelerated aging and disease and thereby improve the quality of your life.

Diana Schwarzbein, M.D.
Santa Barbara, California

PART I

Aging

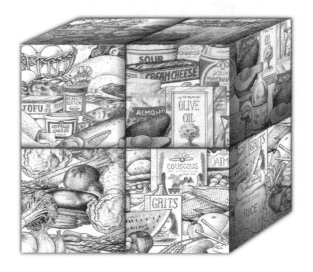

One

What Is the Accelerated Metabolic Aging Process?

W e are all going to age and die, because it is impossible to stop normal aging. But you have more control over aging than you might believe. In fact, you can improve your metabolism, look and feel younger, achieve your ideal body composition and delay the degenerative diseases of aging by simply avoiding the habits that accelerate the normal aging process.

Before reading the patient interviews[1] throughout this book, which explore the degenerative diseases of accelerated metabolic aging in further detail, you must understand what metabolic aging means and how certain habits accelerate this process. As you learn about the accelerated metabolic aging process, you will understand what you can do to heal your metabolism, which in turn will improve your quality of life and increase your longevity.

What Is Metabolism?

In popular terminology, metabolism is defined as the amount of energy a person's body burns. However, burning energy is only a small

---

[1]*Some of the names of the patients mentioned throughout the book have been changed to protect their privacy.*

fraction of what your metabolism does. Metabolism is the combined effects of all the varied biochemical processes that continually occur in your body on a cellular level. These processes enable every individual component of your body to function, making it possible for you to think, digest food, move and perform all the functions of a living, breathing being. Some of these functions include: bone and tissue regeneration, elimination, fertility, functions of all internal organs, mood, vision, hormone production, heart pumping and talking.

Regeneration processes are divided into two categories: Those that build the body up and those that break the body down. Your body is made up of dynamic tissues such as nails and hair that your body constantly replaces. This breaking-down process is essential for clearing out the old cells and cellular material (enzymes, hormones, neurotransmitters) to make room for the new.

Aging and Hormones

Hormones are the chemical communicators within your body that direct the cellular building processes. Hormones, and the messages they send, are essential for breaking down old cells and making new cells. Likewise, healthy new cells are important for hormone production. When a particular hormone system breaks down, as with the loss of estrogen from the ovaries, it affects all the other processes in the entire physiological system because the systems of the body are interconnected. As your body loses cells and hormone levels decline, your body breaks down more than it builds up, and the end result is aging.

Cellular Aging

To explain, in simple terms, how cells age, I will focus on two types of cells: stem cells and committed cells.

Stem cells have one purpose: to produce committed cells. Under the direction of various hormones, stem cells divide slowly over the course of your lifetime to make new stem cells.

Committed cells perform all the biochemical processes of your metabolism. These cells are short-lived; they are constantly being replaced by new committed cells.

With the normal wear and tear of time, your stem cells wear down and produce fewer and less-efficient committed cells. As your committed cells continue to decrease and become less efficient, your body breaks down more than it builds up. Because there are fewer and fewer committed cells available, and because more of them are less efficient, your metabolism (your body's ability to carry out chemical and other processes) goes into a decline.

If your stem cells continued to produce an adequate supply of perfect committed cells, your metabolism would not age and you would not age. Your vitality and health would never decline. But the decreased efficiency of your metabolism is the natural and inevitable result of cellular aging.

In summary, normal cellular aging is a cycle that goes like this: Stem cells make committed cells, committed cells make hormones, hormones direct the stem cells to make more committed cells, and so on. Normal cellular aging results as committed cells die but do not get replaced, or are replaced with less efficient committed cells. Because, ultimately, our bodies will be made up of both stem cells and committed cells that are imperfect or that have been damaged by a variety of factors (aging, free radicals, radiation, toxins, prolonged high insulin levels and so on), we will all age and die. There is no way to prevent *normal* cellular aging.

Accelerated Metabolic Aging

Due to various genetic differences, everyone is programmed to live a certain number of years. Achieving your individual maximum life expectancy requires that you maintain a healthy, functioning metabolism. However, when unhealthy eating and lifestyle habits interfere with hormone production, the metabolic system breaks down faster than normal. This premature breakdown is what I call "accelerated metabolic aging."

Naturally, if you are aging rapidly on the cellular level, you are going to look older and feel older much faster.

Though you cannot change *normal* metabolic aging, you do have control over *accelerated* metabolic aging. In fact, it is possible to stop and even heal some of the damage done to your body by the accelerated metabolic aging process. Some nutrition and lifestyle habits that can accelerate this process are shown in the box below.

Nutrition and Lifestyle Habits That Accelerate Metabolic Aging

Alcohol
Artificial sweeteners
Caffeine
Excessive and/or unnecessary thyroid replacement therapy
Lack of exercise
Poor nutrition
Prescription or over-the-counter drug use[2]
Steroids
Stimulant and other recreational drugs
Stress
Tobacco

Insulin Resistance

Over the course of the normal aging process, everyone develops what is called insulin resistance. It is normal for a ninety-year-old

---

[2] *All drugs, over-the-counter and prescription, adversely affect your metabolism. This does not mean that you should stop taking your prescribed medication. You should, however, be aware, and circumspect, about everything that goes into your body.*

person to be insulin resistant. However, because of accelerated metabolic aging, people are developing insulin resistance at much younger ages: forty, thirty and even twenty-five.

Benjamin was a perfect example of someone who was insulin resistant. At age fifty-six, a routine blood panel showed the red flag of high blood sugar. His story illustrates a case of accelerated metabolic aging.

Benjamin: My wife and I moved to Santa Barbara five years ago. I was already at an advanced stage of degenerative arthritis in my hips. In the summer of 1992 I had one hip replaced, and the next summer I was told I needed the other hip replaced. During preparation for the second hip surgery, my rheumatologist noticed that my blood-sugar level was above the acceptable range. He suggested that I see Diana Schwarzbein. When I went to see her, I had high blood sugar and high blood pressure, my cholesterol level was too high and, most important, I had gained a lot of weight despite every effort to keep my fat intake under control.

Dr. Schwarzbein: Benjamin was suffering from the conditions he listed because he had developed insulin resistance at an early age. I explained to him that insulin is a hormone and that hormones are the chemical communicators between all cells. All hormones depend on each other to do their jobs. For the body to function well, all hormones must be kept at normal levels. Just as it is not healthy to have high or low thyroid levels or high or low estrogen levels, it is not healthy to have high or low insulin levels. You do not want high or low hormone levels; you want normal hormone levels interacting with one another. When your hormone levels are normal, we say they are balanced.

The hormone insulin's major function is to regulate blood-sugar levels, thereby protecting the brain from receiving too much sugar, which damages cells. As you read in the Introduction,[3] insulin accomplishes this in two ways: First, the presence of insulin alerts the liver to incoming high amounts of sugar so that the liver does not let this high sugar pass

---

[3] *If you skipped the Introduction, please return and read it because it contains information that is essential for your total understanding of the concepts in this book.*

through to the brain. Second, insulin stows away sugar into cells, thereby decreasing blood-sugar levels. Think of cells as having locked "doors" and insulin as the *only* key that fits the lock to the doors. Cells have numerous receptors that are the locked doors that insulin opens. After opening these doors, insulin unloads blood sugar to fuel the cells of the body.

This system of checks and balances works well with a balanced diet of proteins, fats, nonstarchy vegetables and carbohydrates. However, the typical diet today is too high in carbohydrates, which means high sugar. Also, over the course of a lifetime your metabolic processes slow down, and your body does not need as many carbohydrates for energy as it did when you were younger. However, many of us still eat the same meals now as we ate ten or twenty years ago. If these meals are high in carbohydrates, we are eating more energy than our metabolism needs today.

Years of high-carbohydrate meals translate into years of excessive cumulative sugar in the body. After many years, cells become so filled with sugar that they cannot admit any more sugar molecules. To protect against further sugar overload, the cells reduce the number of insulin receptors (doors) they have so that insulin will not be able to unload as much sugar. This is insulin resistance. Next, the pancreas secretes even more insulin in an attempt to overcome this resistance. This results in too much insulin in the bloodstream, a condition known as *hyperinsulinemia*. The cells react to the excess insulin by locking even more insulin receptor doors, leading to further insulin resistance. At this stage, any extra sugar in the bloodstream is diverted into fat storage. When the fat cells are filled, the sugar has nowhere to go and remains in the bloodstream. This is Type II diabetes.

Benjamin was caught in this vicious cycle. I explained how he could reverse insulin resistance and thus repair his metabolism through proper nutrition and lifestyle habits.

Benjamin: I have always had a weight problem, but none of my previous doctors ever recommended any specific nutritional program. Throughout my life, I never "dieted," but I did try to keep my caloric intake down and to avoid high-cholesterol foods. My wife was after me to avoid red meat, eggs, and to eat a lot of fresh fruit and vegetables. I based my diet on the kind of conventional wisdom one acquires by reading newspapers and magazines.

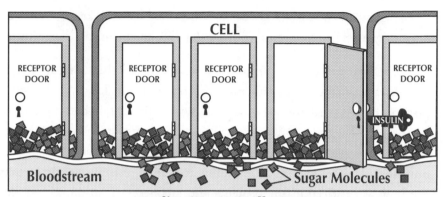

Insulin Opens Cell Doors

Body cells have numerous receptors for insulin. Think of these receptors as doors through which insulin, the key, enables sugar molecules to enter the cell.

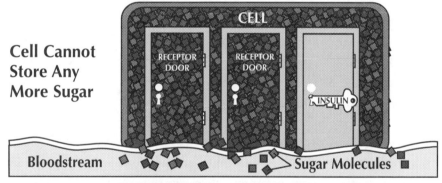

After many years of high carbohydrate consumption, body cells become so filled with energy (sugar) that they can no longer admit additional sugar.

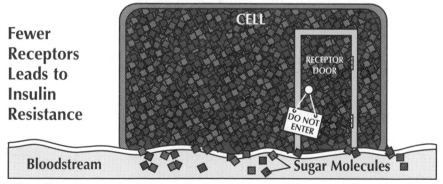

The cells protect against further sugar overload by reducing the number of receptors. The remaining receptors also become more resistant to the actions of insulin.

Figure 1-1. How Insulin Resistance Develops

Dr. Schwarzbein asked me what I had for breakfast and I told her, "Typically, a bowl of cold cereal with low-fat milk and a glass of orange juice."

Dr. Schwarzbein: Benjamin's breakfast of cereal with low-fat milk and orange juice is a typical low-fat, high-carbohydrate breakfast. All the components of this meal are carbohydrates, with little protein and no fat.

You have learned about one vicious cycle of insulin resistance, when cells become overloaded with sugar and refuse to allow insulin to unload any more. Another vicious cycle leading to insulin resistance occurs when the body is deprived of the proteins and fats necessary to build muscle. Muscle is filled with cells that have insulin receptor doors. Therefore, less muscle mass equals fewer insulin receptor doors, which contributes to insulin resistance.

Over the years, Benjamin's body's need for energy decreased, but he continued to eat too many carbohydrates. A closer look at his body composition showed he had increased his body fat by eating an excess of carbohydrates and decreased his lean muscle mass by depriving his body of protein and fats. This occurred because muscle mass is made from the proteins and fats we eat. Carbohydrates do not build muscle. As Benjamin's muscle mass was depleted, his muscle cell doors were depleted as well, which meant fewer doors for insulin to unload blood sugar through. But early on, the fat cells can accommodate excess sugar. With his muscle mass depleted, more and more of Benjamin's carbohydrates were converted into fat and stored into fat cells around his middle. I call the fat deposition around the midsection the "insulin meter" because this is an area where insulin first deposits extra fat. When I see patients with an excess of body fat around their midsections, I immediately know they have an insulin imbalance.

Benjamin: Dr. Schwarzbein suggested that I lower my carbohydrate intake for a short period of time and eat more proteins, fats and non-starchy vegetables. What she said to me made sense, and I was at a point in my life where I was feeling a little desperate.

Dr. Schwarzbein: I asked Benjamin to go on the same healing program that I developed while working with Type II diabetics, which includes eating more fats and reducing carbohydrate consumption. I explained that eating fat would not make him fat. Fat cannot be stored without the presence of insulin because insulin is necessary to store fat in fat cells. Fats do not stimulate insulin secretion at all. Even if a person ate fat all day long, this would not stimulate the pancreas to secrete insulin; therefore fat could not be stored in the fat cells.[4]

The healing program is prescribed for people who have been overdoing carbohydrates, like Benjamin, and who have seriously damaged their health and metabolism. During the initial stages of the healing program, I ask patients to decrease their carbohydrate consumption slightly below their current metabolic needs and, instead, to eat more proteins, fats and nonstarchy vegetables.[5] This allows their body to begin to heal by using their stored sugar. As cells become emptied of sugar, they replace the insulin receptor doors that had previously been closed to insulin. This is a reversal of insulin resistance, and patients are on their way to reversing accelerated metabolic aging.

The length of time you need to spend on the nutritional healing program is determined by your present state of health. The more you have indulged in eating and lifestyle habits that accelerate metabolic aging, the longer you will need to be in the healing phase. But the healing program is not meant to continue for the rest of your life.

Once your symptoms or illnesses are corrected, the maintenance program will prevent the same problems from recurring or new problems from developing. The maintenance program is also for *healthy* adults and children who want to prevent illnesses.

Benjamin: My first reaction to the diet was, does this mean I have to give up wine? I happen to enjoy a good glass of wine. Dr. Schwarzbein said that I could make tradeoffs in what I ate.

---

[4] *Any food, however, can be stored as fat if there are insulin stimulating factors present: Eating a low-fat, high-carbohydrate diet, stress, dieting, caffeine, alcohol, aspartame, tobacco, steroids, stimulant and other recreational drugs, lack of exercise, excessive and/or unnecessary thyroid replacement therapy and all over-the-counter and prescription drugs.*

[5] *It is extremely important to note that no one should ever go on a zero-carbohydrate diet, because this leads to many hormone imbalances and accelerates metabolic aging.*

Dr. Schwarzbein: Alcohol is a double-edged sword; it is a combination of alcohol and sugar. The alcohol poisons cells and the sugar raises insulin levels. I explained to Benjamin that if drinking a glass of wine relieves stress, then it is better to have that glass of wine than to have the stress. On the other hand, if a person drinks to excess to relieve stress, it is better to have the stress!

The best drink is water. I ask my patients to drink ten eight-ounce glasses of water every day. Since 40 to 50 percent of our body is made up of water, and since water is involved in numerous metabolic functions, drinking water is essential if you want to be healthy.

Benjamin: Other than wine, how would I feel about giving up things that I had always considered essential in my life? I was raised by an immigrant mother whose idea of a healthy meal was a lot of starch. The idea of living without potatoes, rice or pasta, pizza or lots of bread was very off-putting at first. On the other hand, I was lucky that some items on this diet are allowed without restriction, like eggs, meat, poultry and fish.

I consider myself very lucky that on this eating program I can keep my blood-sugar levels, my cholesterol levels and my weight down. This is important to me because I have a family history of diabetes. I am fifty-nine and my father acquired diabetes sometime in his sixties, so clearly I am at risk.

Dr. Schwarzbein: As Benjamin said, there is a risk factor for diabetes in his family. But that risk factor is not purely genetic. It is mostly acquired. Benjamin is from a family whose "idea of a healthy meal was a lot of starch." Family members usually share the same diet and lifestyle habits, so they generally have the same risk factors.

Degenerative Diseases Are Not Genetic but Acquired

As you learned earlier, insulin is a hormone, and all hormones communicate with each other. Increased insulin levels disrupt every other hormone system in the body. For example, high insulin levels in women lead to increased testosterone levels, which then blunt estrogen effects which can then lead to no ovulation and decreased progesterone production. Or increased insulin leads to increased adrenaline and cortisol levels, which means that you now have three hormone levels increased out of normal ranges. Over time, hormone imbalances always lead to disease.

When insulin levels are kept high too long, the result is a physiology that promotes excessive body-fat gain, a physiology prone to infections and all the chronic degenerative diseases of aging: osteoarthritis, different types of cancer, cholesterol abnormalities, coronary artery disease, less lean body mass[6] with excess body fat, high blood pressure, osteoporosis, stroke and Type II diabetes.

The medical establishment considers these degenerative diseases to be genetically transmitted. Again, I disagree. Consider the following: Genetic diseases manifest themselves and are diagnosed in childhood or early adolescence. Excessive body-fat gain and decreased lean body mass, as well as the diseases listed above, occur primarily in adults and are usually manifested after age thirty.

By the time you are thirty years old, your cells do not utilize sugar as well as they did when you were younger; this is cellular aging. But time is not the only factor that causes cellular aging. What you have eaten and how you have lived your life will determine the actual age of your cells, and therefore the health of your metabolism at any given time. In other words, even though all thirty-year-olds are the same chronological age, they are different metabolic ages.

High insulin levels are also considered genetic. But the majority of people are not born with too much insulin. People acquire prolonged high insulin levels primarily through aging, stress, dieting, caffeine, alcohol, tobacco, steroids, lack of exercise, stimulant and other recreational drugs, excessive and/or unnecessary thyroid replacement

---

[6] In this text, lean body mass refers to muscle and bone mass.

therapy, all over-the-counter and prescription drugs and, most important, eating a diet deficient in proteins and fats while eating excess carbohydrates.

Of course, as you read earlier, there are genetic variables. The example used in the Introduction, which I will repeat here, was that of insulin response. Everyone (except Type I diabetics) secretes a different amount of insulin in response to the same amount of carbohydrates. However, this is clinically significant only when eating and lifestyle habits consistently cause insulin levels to rise. If everyone ate a balanced diet of real foods[7] and avoided stimulants and stress, there would be no appreciable difference between those people who secreted more insulin and those who did not. Another example of a genetic variable might be a person's response to stress. Even though the same stress hormones are released in response to stress, the amount can vary. Those whose bodies secrete higher levels of hormones in response to stress will, in the long run, age faster.

But this book is not about all the exceptions that can occur in individuals. This book is about making positive eating and lifestyle changes to improve your metabolism, regardless of your individual genetic differences. The choice is yours. You can resign yourself to your genetic predisposition or you can alter your personal physiology through positive eating and lifestyle changes. As you learned in the Introduction, the way to prevent aging and to promote good health and weight loss is by first focusing on this principle: *Degenerative diseases are not genetic but acquired. Because the systems of the human body are interconnected and because one imbalance creates another imbalance, poor eating and lifestyle habits, not genetics, are the major causes of degenerative disease.* I hope that you will choose to make positive changes that will promote balance and improve the quality of your life!

---

[7] *Because manufacturers have misused the word "natural" in advertising their invented foods and adulterated food products, people do not understand what natural means anymore. For that reason I have reeducated my patients to eat only "real" foods which they could, in theory, pick, gather, milk, hunt or fish. For example, an egg is a real food, but chemical egg substitutes are not.*

Prolonged high insulin levels brought on by bad eating and lifestyle habits age the metabolism on a cellular level. This aging process leads to disease. In other words, illness and accelerated metabolic aging are outcomes of the same process. Anyone's metabolism can be ruined by diet and lifestyle, causing that person to become ill. Understanding that disease is a late indicator of metabolic aging is key to understanding why degenerative diseases are not genetic but acquired.

Benjamin: Four years ago, I went on the healing program full time with the carbohydrate quotas and working out on a stationary bicycle on a daily basis. In six months I lost thirty pounds and four inches off of my waistline which I have not regained. It cost me a small fortune to have my wardrobe redone.

All the indicators that suggested I was at risk for full-blown diabetes have remained stable or improved—blood pressure, cholesterol, weight and blood sugar.

I don't crave the things that I thought I was going to crave. I remember with fondness pizza or big pieces of fudge cake, but I no longer feel any active craving for them. I haven't lived an unhappy life for four years thinking about these things. For the most part, I am very comfortable with this way of eating.

My weight leveled off after six months. Since that time I have added a few pounds of muscle due to the fact that I have been working with a fitness trainer for the past few years.

Dr. Schwarzbein: Throughout this book you will read interviews with patients who have suffered from chronic conditions and diseases as a result of accelerated aging brought on by prolonged high insulin levels. The box that follows shows some of the chronic conditions and degenerative diseases that are covered in this book.

Damage Caused by Prolonged
High Insulin in the Human Body

Acne

Addictions

Asthma

Cancer (rapid cell growth)

Carbohydrate and stimulant
   craving

Delayed puberty

Depression and mood swings

Eating disorders

Excessive weight gain

Heartburn and other
   gastrointestinal disorders

Heart disease (plaqueing of
   the coronary arteries)

High cholesterol and
   triglyceride levels

Infertility

Insomnia and fatigue

Insulin resistance, leading
   eventually to Type II diabetes

Irritable bowel syndrome

Low estrogen

Migraine headaches

Osteoporosis

In summary, aging is a normal process and insulin resistance is a normal phenomenon of aging. Degenerative diseases are not genetic but result from all the eating and lifestyle habits that accelerate metabolic aging. If you do your best to maintain normal insulin levels, you will delay insulin resistance and slow down the aging process significantly. In turn, the habits that normalize insulin levels normalize all other hormone systems as well. Keeping hormone levels balanced is the key to preventing degenerative diseases and to extending longevity.

Again, one primary goal in avoiding accelerated metabolic aging is to avoid developing insulin resistance for as long as possible. Dietary fat is vital to delaying insulin resistance and preventing accelerated metabolic aging. The following chapter explains why.

Two

Human Survival Depends on Hormones and Fat

The balanced eating program I prescribe for my patients is appropriate for everyone because we all share the same physiology (the physical and chemical processes that define humans as the same species). The DNA (genetic blueprint), biochemistry and endocrinology of human beings has not changed in millions of years.

In prehistoric times, survival of the fittest meant surviving infectious diseases such as viruses, parasites and bacteria, as well as avoiding accidents and escaping violent death. In addition, humans were susceptible to inborn errors of metabolism (such as a five-year-old child dying of heart disease), autoimmune diseases (such as Type I diabetes), genetic defects (such as sickle-cell anemia) and the normal aging process. All of these things were beyond human control.

The average life expectancy of a prehistoric human was eighteen to twenty-five years. Most died of infectious diseases such as pneumonia. Those who had the most developed hormone systems survived the longest because a developed hormone system is essential for a strong immune system. Since a lack of hormones leads to a weakened immune system, many died young and most did not survive past midlife. Children and adults past midlife were the most susceptible to viruses and bacteria, because children's hormone systems were not developed fully and older adults had diminished hormone systems.

In modern times, we have eradicated most plagues with immunizations. We now prevent bacteria from multiplying through the use of antibiotics, sanitation, refrigeration and food preservatives. Today most people do not die of infectious diseases but of degenerative diseases. Therefore, *avoiding the accelerated metabolic aging process in modern times is the new definition of survival of the fittest.*

Modern humans still have the same physiology as prehistoric humans, and this physiology depends on proteins and fats to produce hormones and regulate them. How you balance your hormones throughout your life will affect your life span. Hormone regulation is within your control.

Since hormones, including insulin, depend on fat for normal production and functioning, eating fat is essential for our survival.

Wasting Away on a Low-Fat Diet

I have seen many patients who appeared to be suffering from either cancer or AIDS. When I started asking these patients about their habits, it did not take long to discover why they were wasting away. By the time Robert came to see me, I had learned to tell the difference between real disease and self-imposed (though not intentional) starvation.

Robert, an articulate, dignified man in his late sixties, came to me at his wife's urging. His wife, Linda, had heard me speak on menopause and nutrition, and she made an appointment with me to discuss her issues. As I got to know her, I learned that she was worried about her husband, who had suffered two heart attacks. During one appointment, I asked Linda how Robert was doing. She burst into tears. When I learned that Robert was eating an extreme low-fat diet, I gave him a call and asked him to come in to see me.

Robert: I had my first heart attack when I was sixty years old. I was not ready to die, so my wife and I read every one of Nathan Pritikin's books, and one book written by his son. I went on the Pritikin Diet to improve my cholesterol profile.

In an attempt to rid my diet of fat, I started to eat only sixteen ounces of protein (meat, fish or poultry) a week and gradually reduced it to four ounces a week. The balance of my diet consisted of vegetables, with a heavy emphasis on carbohydrates—grains, beans, pastas and fruits. Almost no fat. I did not add fat to anything. I'm a type A personality. I'm disciplined, persistent and tenacious about things. I did not do the Pritikin Diet halfway. I did what Pritikin said to do. I mean, my wife and I were in the kitchen measuring, going through all this math computation about fat and everything else.

I had suffered from gastrointestinal problems for some time and they were getting worse. The reflux and spasms increased in frequency and severity. I had very uncomfortable gas. I would have chest pains and wouldn't know if I was having a heart attack or esophageal spasms. I can't tell you how many times I went to the emergency room because I thought I was having another heart attack, only to be told it was reflux again.

Then, six years later, in June of 1992, I did have another heart attack and had to have heart bypass surgery. After the lengths I had gone to, to minimize fats in my diet, I was told that I had three blood vessels clogged! I thought, *How could this be?* I had exercised and done every-thing by the book.

After the surgery, I went on Pritikin's total vegetarian diet.

During this time I became so fatigued that I could do very little. The energy I did have was spent going to doctors and desperately reading medical literature to try to determine what was wrong with me. The doc-tors had nothing to offer except test after test and acid-blocking drugs. One doctor concluded that I was depressed, and he wanted me to take antidepressants, which I refused to do. Another concluded that I was a hypochondriac.

I went from 155 pounds in 1992 to 139 pounds by late 1994. I am five feet, ten inches so, at 155 pounds, I was already very thin.

I was not sleeping well at all. I was up most nights with heartburn, stomach and chest pains. One such night I was up until four in the morning with chest pains. My wife called 911 and took me to a hospital emergency room. Again, it was determined that I was not having a heart attack. The cardiologist and gastroenterologist, working together, ran tests on about every organ of my body. The upshot of all the tests and examinations was in essence, "Gee, we don't know what's making you sick."

I didn't know what else to do at that point. Then I got a call from Dr. Schwarzbein, who had spoken to my wife. After that conversation, I visited Dr. Schwarzbein to see if she could improve my cholesterol profile and perhaps prevent another heart attack.

Dr. Schwarzbein: I was shocked when I first saw Robert. The extreme low-fat diet that he was on had aged him inside and out by depriving his body of the important nutrients it needed to regenerate.

By eating a high-carbohydrate diet, Robert had sustained prolonged high insulin levels, which in turn disrupted other hormone levels, causing heartburn and other gastrointestinal problems and an abnormal cholesterol profile. We had to reverse the process immediately because Robert was in the danger zone. He was going to die if he stayed on his low-fat, low-protein, high-carbohydrate diet.

I explained to Robert that hormones are made from and regulated by the proteins and fats we eat. Therefore, to maintain normal body-system communication and repair and rebuilding, we must eat a balanced diet that includes proteins and fats.

As you learned in the previous chapter, regeneration can be described as the combined effects of all the processes that build the body up, plus those that break it down. We need to eat to replenish cellular resources and energy stores for all the processes within the body. Eating increases metabolism. When you break your body down more than you build it up, you lower your metabolism. This is accelerated metabolic aging. Again, this aging process leads to disease. Because illness and accelerated metabolic aging are outcomes of the same process, anyone's metabolism can be ruined by diet and lifestyle, causing that person to become ill.

Many people do not understand that eating is essential to life. I explained to Robert that the body functions to keep the brain alive and protect it from harm. There are two sources of raw materials available to keep the brain alive and to fuel the continual reconstruction that goes on within your body:

1. Food: Each time you take a bite of food, you have a new opportunity to change your metabolism. By eating the right foods, you not only ensure your survival; you improve your health, too.

2. Your own body mass: If you eat less than adequate amounts of food or the wrong combination of foods, you will consume your own tissue stores to stay alive. Needless to say, if you had no food at all you would eventually die. Indeed, people are slowly killing themselves on a daily basis by depriving their bodies of essential raw materials. They are, in effect, eating themselves from the inside out.

I will take you through the process of the low-fat, low-calorie diet that I described to Robert so you can understand why this form of dieting causes the body to go into survival mode and waste away.

Low-Fat, Low-Calorie Diets Turn Off Your Metabolism

1. Your liver stores a twelve-hour supply of ready energy called glycogen. When you go on a low-fat, low-calorie diet, your body initially uses this stored liver glycogen in lieu of enough food to maintain tightly regulated blood-sugar levels going to the brain.

2. At the same time that the brain is tapping into the liver glycogen stores, the muscles are using their own glycogen stores for locomotion. Initial weight loss from a calorie-restricted diet can be substantial as your body burns up its muscle glycogen stores, because glycogen is sugar stored with water and is therefore heavy. But since these ready stores of energy are in short supply, your weekly weight loss quickly begins to plateau.

"Water Weight"

When people say, "I've lost water weight," it's true.

Glycogen is the human carbohydrate. It is made up of chains of sugar molecules hooked up together with water molecules. Since water is heavy, carbohydrates are an inefficient form for storing energy. Fat molecules (triglycerides) do not contain water, so they are much lighter than carbohydrates and are a more efficient way to store energy. Your body can store more than twice as much energy as fat than it can as carbohydrates in the same amount of weight. A 160-pound man with 20 percent body fat would weigh 192 pounds if his fat stores were converted to carbohydrate stores.

In the early stages of a calorie-restricted diet, glycogen stores are used up and the water generated, when glycogen is broken down into sugar, is lost through urination. Because glycogen weighs so much more than fat, low-calorie diets can result in a weight loss of up to nine pounds in the first week. This is the reason low-calorie diets show immediate results; but these results are not sustained over time.

---

3. When the liver glycogen stores are depleted, your liver turns your structural proteins into sugar for brain utilization. Fats (triglycerides) cannot be used for brain fuel.

4. Proteins and fats are necessary for metabolic processes and the constant rebuilding that must go on within your body. When you cut back on dietary fats and proteins, your body is forced to take these materials from bones and muscles to keep up the rebuilding processes. It is like trying to build a home without all the materials. You must continually tear down one room to build another. This is a metabolic disaster.

5. During this period of undernourishment, your body will burn some fat for energy. But fat loss is minimal compared to the

destruction that is happening to your muscle and bone mass. You are losing more weight by depleting muscle and bone mass than you are from burning the fat as energy.

6. Obviously your body cannot continue indefinitely to use its muscle and bone mass, because muscle and bone are both needed to function as structural body parts. So your body begins to slow down your metabolic processes to stop the consumption of your body tissues.

7. Taking care of the brain cells that maintain major body functions, such as breathing, is your body's first priority, so the brain keeps feeding off the body. All other systems continue to slow. If there is only enough protein from your own muscle and bone-mass stores for the brain to accomplish very basic functions, you will become tired. This fatigue is a good indicator that the body is not getting what it needs. At this point, if you do not get off the low-calorie, low-fat diet and start eating a more balanced diet, you will begin to experience the initial symptoms of malnutrition: worsening fatigue, dry skin, thinning hair and nails, irregular menstrual periods, loss of memory and the inability to concentrate, loss of muscle mass and tone, depression and loss of sexual interest.

8. As your body gets less and less of what it needs, it continues to waste away. All your body can do is try to slow down its systems further in order to conserve energy. The body perceives this famine as an extremely dangerous situation because at this point the body is starving. It shuts down even further in order to save itself; and, like Robert, you will experience the warning symptoms that something is wrong. (Of course if the famine continued, the last stage would be death.)

In Robert's case, all of the above added up to significant amounts of weight loss and a myriad of chronic conditions and illnesses. He was literally eating himself up. When the body uses itself for resources, you are in the process of dying, not living. Building up is living. Breaking down is dying. Robert was breaking down. As he wasted away, he felt and looked like a very old man. As he starved his body, it broke down entirely.

In an effort to do the right thing, Robert had adopted a radically low-fat diet that reset his metabolism to an extremely low state and accelerated his metabolic aging process. He persisted in what his body perceived as a famine, and this famine went on for an extended period of time until Robert's body suffered from malnutrition.

Why We Need Protein

One of the most dangerous aspects of the low-fat movement is low-protein intake. Like Robert, if you decrease the amount of fats you eat, then you are likely to decrease the amount of proteins too because many proteins and fats occur together in nature. Eggs, red meat and nuts are a few examples.

Proteins are comprised of amino acids. There are twenty amino acids that are important for human metabolism. Ten of these amino acids can be produced within the body and are called nonessential. The other ten, which are required for life but not made in the body, are called essential amino acids; these must be obtained by eating protein.

Humans need a steady source of protein for the constant rebuilding that goes on within the body, including hormone production. Without protein the body ceases to regenerate, and hormone production declines and/or becomes imbalanced.

Proteins called immunoglobulins are the substance of your immune system. Without these proteins, you weaken your immune system. So when people try to reduce fat by cutting protein, their immune systems are greatly compromised. This was the case with Robert.

I knew that the healing program would be a shock to Robert, given what he had been doing all those years. I had to get his attention fast and help him to take a good look at himself. I told him he looked like a very old man—ninety-something, not sixty-something—and that if I had not known better I might have thought he had AIDS or was dying of cancer. I also assured him that the healing program would also cure his heartburn. Heartburn is the burning sensation felt when acid from the stomach rises back up the esophagus. When you think about eating, your body assumes it will receive protein, and your stomach produces hydrochloric acid. The purpose of this acid is to activate enzymes for the digestion of proteins. On a low-fat, low-protein diet, the carbohydrates you eat go through the stomach so quickly that the outpouring of acid has nowhere to go but up. To complicate the issue, later on, insulin, stimulated by these carbohydrates, further increases acid production by activating other hormone systems.

Dr. Schwarzbein: By this point in my clinical practice I had found that the more good fats people eat, the healthier they become. But I felt that if I shared this with Robert, it might scare him away from even considering the healing program. Instead, I asked him to eat proteins and fats with every meal. I explained that nutritional requirements are the same for everyone—a balanced diet from the four nutrient groups: proteins, fats, nonstarchy vegetables and carbohydrates.

I saw the doubt in Robert's eyes that first visit. He may not have been at all receptive to this program at an earlier time in his life because of his conviction that a low-fat diet was healthy. But he did not know what else to do. He had stuck to a strict low-fat, vegetarian diet, using mathematical tables and scales in a heroic effort to save his own life. He had followed the low-fat program religiously and ended up with coronary-artery bypass surgery.

Robert: When Dr. Schwarzbein told me about her eating program, I was very skeptical. I am a conservative person and not inclined to go off on a tangent. I carefully considered the program and finally concluded that it was worth a try.

I started eating tuna and reintroduced meat and chicken into my diet. I ate peanut butter again and hard-boiled eggs, vegetables, of course, fish, fowl, meat, cheese, mayonnaise, some fruit, and a little bit of other carbo-hydrates, like rice.

I regained weight and am now 155 pounds again. I do not suffer from heartburn, reflux or spasms of the esophagus. My gas, stomach pains, constipation and diarrhea have all disappeared. My cholesterol numbers are normal. And—very important—my energy has returned. For the first time in many years I feel like I am living, not dying. I understand now that I was literally starving myself to death on the Pritikin Diet.

Dr. Schwarzbein: Once convinced to try the program, Robert applied the same commitment that he had with the low-fat diet. Over the last two years, he has improved dramatically. At seventy, he looks and feels healthier than he has in many years. He will continue to improve as his body becomes nourished. Restoring proteins and fats gave Robert's cells the nutrients they needed to balance hormones, begin to reverse insulin resistance, heal his metabolism and get off the accelerated metabolic aging track.

You may not have taken the low-fat diet to the same extreme as Robert did. But do you go hungry much of the time? Are you fatigued, not sleeping well? Do you have heartburn and other intestinal problems? Low-fat dieting promises health but instead makes you unhealthy. Even if you are overweight, if you are eating a low-fat diet you are starving your body. Every day that you eat a low-fat diet, your metabolism slows down.

Our bodies are incredible machines that can withstand a lot of internal stresses and still keep us alive. But just being alive is not good enough. Quality of life is important, and you will not have a quality life or a quality body from a diet that upsets the nutritional balance the human body needs.

The good news is that lifelong metabolism is a dynamic process. Metabolism is resilient: It is shaped by past and present input. Basic tenets of the physiology of the metabolism do not change. Your response to foods may be affected by genetics to a certain degree, but the way in which we all process foods is the same. This is what I mean when I say we all have the same physiology.

Like many people, Robert did not know that fat is one of the important nutrients for human survival. Without fat, you will die much more quickly. This is because fats constitute a large part of your body, not as unwanted pounds but as cell membranes, hormones and other vital structures.

No matter what else a person does, low-fat dieting dramatically compounds damage to his or her metabolism because virtually eliminating two essential nutrient groups upsets the balance that the human body needs for constant nourishment. Low-fat dieting accelerates insulin resistance and aging, which leads to degenerative diseases.

The fact that humans have a resilient metabolism is why, with balanced nutrition, it was possible for Robert to reverse the accelerated metabolic aging process and restore his health. But low-fat dieting is not the only threat to human survival, as you will learn in chapter 3.

Three

Humans Are Part of
the Food Chain

Since the Industrial Revolution, most people have stopped picking, gathering, milking, hunting or fishing for their foods. People now eat invented, chemically altered or created substances we call "food products." We tend to think that our bodies will simply process anything we put in them. But every single thing that goes into our mouths should be used as building material or energy. If it is not, our bodies perceive it as a dangerous substance. Products like saccharin, margarine and other invented substances, along with refined and processed foods, are harmful because they damage cells. Because chemical processes proceed on a molecular level, we must think about what we put into our bodies. In fact, since we have personally stopped picking, gathering, milking, hunting or fishing for our food, we must think even more about what we ingest.

Perhaps we no longer think about the various chemicals we ingest—in the form of processed foods, invented foods and other nonfood items—because we do not understand the *biological* food chain. I believe that once people understand the food chain, they will no longer consume the same chemicals and nonfoods without fearing for their health.

In simplified terms, the food chain depends on the transfer of energy in the environment from one system to another. Humans, like all living things, are made up of essential elements—oxygen, hydrogen, nitrogen and carbon (to name a few). These elements get recycled from the earth to us through the foods we eat and the air we breathe. In turn, when we die, we return these elements to the soil. To break it down even further:

1. The sun gives energy to the plants in the form of solar heat.

2. The solar energy, along with fertilizer, rich in nutrients, enable plants to grow and produce oxygen as a by-product (photosynthesis).

3. Animals breathe the air and graze on the plants and are nourished. Some animals have the enzymatic ability to digest cellulose into sugar and convert it to protein to replenish their bodies. This is how elements from plants are transferred to the tissues of the animals.

4. Since humans do not have the ability to digest cellulose into replenishing proteins, animals, lower on the food chain, provide that nourishment (proteins) in the form of meat and dairy products for humans.

5. Humans, animals and plants die and decompose, leaving nutrients in the soil as fertilizer.

6. The cycle continues.

We humans, as living beings, are made up of dynamic tissues, such as nails and hair, that are constantly being replaced. This breaking-down process is essential for clearing out the old cells and cellular material (enzymes, hormones, neurotransmitters) to make room for the new. This regeneration process is made possible by the fact that we eat the very same biochemicals of which we are inherently composed. In other words, we are made up of the same elements as those in the plants and animals we eat. We are not made up of the elements that go into nonfoods and other substances that are not found in nature.

If we could see with the naked eye the intricate biochemical processes going on within our bodies, we would be appalled at the damage we do to ourselves when we ingest chemicals. For example, if after drinking a diet soda we could actually see what occurs on a cellular level—how the molecules, hormones and enzymes become imbalanced—it would be apparent that such a substance is bad for our bodies. But because the damage happens out of sight, we continue to travel along the accelerated metabolic aging track, and our health deteriorates slowly over a long period of time. Then when we gain body fat or have a health crisis, it seems as though the problem manifested itself suddenly.

The biological food chain has been altered in a devastating way by the Industrial Revolution. We now rely on invented technologies to manufacture the food products we eat, and many people automatically assume that these substances are healthy to consume. But the introduction of chemicals as food—instead of eating real food—has harmed human beings at the cellular level, resulting in accelerated metabolic aging and earlier chronic degenerative diseases. This insidious development now forms a weak link in the food chain: By harming ourselves, we in turn harm the food chain by disrupting nature's balance.

One of the primary goals of this book is to motivate you to stop putting chemicals in your body. I have heard people remark, "Okay, then I won't smoke marijuana." On one hand, I am happy if people can quit at least one destructive habit. I want to encourage you to do whatever you can to become healthier and more aware of your body. On the other hand, I want you to understand that there is no appreciable difference to the human body, between, say, marijuana and aspartame (an artificial sweetener). Any ingested chemicals that are not made in the body damage the body. To your body, the only difference between marijuana, the chemical, and aspartame, the chemical, is the time each takes to destroy the human body on a cellular level.

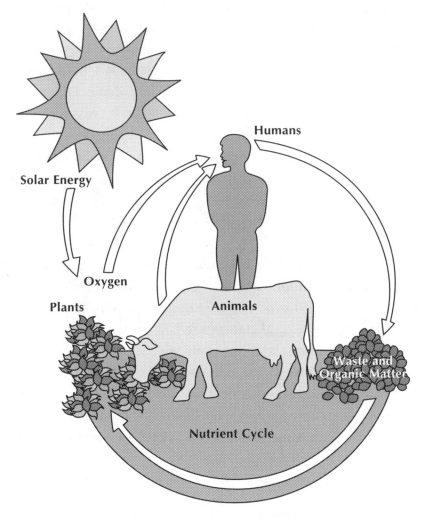

Figure 3-1. The Food Chain

Free Radicals

Any exposure to chemicals—whether ingested, inhaled or absorbed through your skin pores—results in free radicals being introduced into your system. Free radicals are molecules with an extra electron. Since electrons must be paired, these molecules roam your body trying to pair with other electrons by stealing other electrons from your tissues. As a result, free radicals damage the system on a cellular level.

Some free radicals are generated by cigarette smoke, processed fats, exhaust, hairspray, insecticides, sugar and aspartame. In addition, free radicals are created in our bodies during normal metabolism of food. Free radicals are constantly being neutralized in a healthy body by natural antioxidants (vitamins, for example) provided by your diet. The problem arises when, instead of eating foods that would provide antioxidants to neutralize free radicals, people eat "food products" that generate even more free radicals.

Humans are not made out of marijuana, aspartame, hydrogenated oils, diet sodas, fat-free potato chips or other processed food products. The human body cannot use margarine to replenish tissues and cells, or for energy. If you do not eat real food, you are not going to be healthy. Your cells rely on proteins and fats in real food to replenish tissues within your body. Without real food you will damage your cells, accelerating the metabolic aging process that leads first to insulin resistance, then to disease and premature death.

If humans step out of the natural food chain, eventually nature's life cycle will continue without us. It is our choice to be a part of nature. Choosing to be a part of the food chain again is one way we humans can restore our collective health.

If my position seems extreme, it is not because I am in an ivory tower passing judgment. Instead, I have seen what a lifetime of eating invented foods and substances, and using stimulants, can do to our health. It may not be what you want to hear (it is certainly not my goal to take enjoyment out of your life), but I *cannot* tell you that it is okay to ingest chemicals or invented food products. The purpose of this book is to give you all the facts and information you need to improve your health and thereby *enhance* the quality of your life. And the fact is that good health is achieved through eating real foods and following an otherwise balanced lifestyle.

The Schwarzbein Nutrient Groups

In school you learned about the four basic food groups: meats, dairy, breads and grains, and fruits and vegetables. The USDA recently reissued an updated food pyramid. But if you follow these new guidelines you will consume an excess of carbohydrates, which will put you on the accelerated metabolic aging track toward insulin resistance, excess body-fat gain and disease.

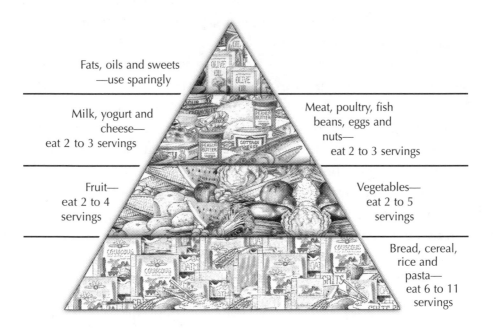

Fats, oils and sweets
—use sparingly

Milk, yogurt and
cheese—
eat 2 to 3 servings

Meat, poultry, fish
beans, eggs and
nuts—
eat 2 to 3 servings

Fruit—
eat 2 to 4
servings

Vegetables—
eat 2 to 5
servings

Bread, cereal,
rice and
pasta—
eat 6 to 11
servings

Figure 3-2. The USDA Food Pyramid

Instead of following the USDA food-group pyramid, which implies a hierarchy of foods, I have designed the Schwarzbein Square as a guide to healthy eating. The square reflects a human physiology dependent on four basic nutrient groups—proteins, fats, nonstarchy vegetables and carbohydrates. In order to survive and thrive we need to eat from all four groups at every meal. Think of it as going back to eating "three squares a day."

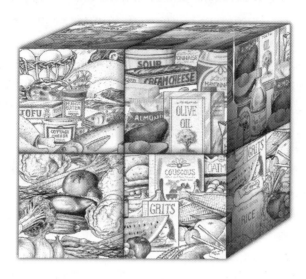

Figure 3-3. The Schwarzbein Square

To keep up the replenishing process within the human body, proteins and fats are the most important of the essential nutrient groups. In addition to making structures (bones, nails, hair), proteins and fats are necessary for the formation of all the chemicals needed for survival, such as hormones, enzymes and neurotransmitters. Nonstarchy vegetables are useful as a source of vitamins, minerals and fiber. Carbohydrates are used mainly to fuel the body, like gasoline for a car. Besides providing these materials and energy, *the four nutrient groups need to be eaten together to balance all the hormone systems of the body.*

The healing-and-maintenance eating programs (explained in detail in Part VIII) are not just one more fad diet that advocates eliminating one or two of the nutrient groups. I am not saying that you should eat only proteins and fats. I am not suggesting that you stop eating carbohydrates, or even drastically reduce carbohydrates in your diet.

This is not a high-fat, high-protein, low-carbohydrate diet. It is a *balanced* nutritional program tailored to improve each individual's specific metabolism. Not eating enough carbohydrates is just as harmful as eating too many. The key to this program is determining your individual carbohydrate need. To do this I am suggesting that *you eat from the four basic nutrient groups* and that you *eat the quantity of real carbohydrates (not man-made) that match your activity level, current health and metabolism.*

Man-made carbohydrates are items such as potato chips, colas, white flour, rice cakes, pasta, bread, cereal and so on. Any carbohydrate that you cannot (at least in theory) pick, gather or milk is man-made. A good example is wheat, which is a real carbohydrate; pasta and bread are man-made. Though you may have recently read that there are "good" carbohydrates and "bad" carbohydrates, there are no "bad" *real* carbohydrates. The only bad carbohydrates are man-made.

Real carbohydrates found in nature are normal stimuli for insulin secretion. However, eating too many real *or* man-made carbohydrates, or ingesting caffeine, tobacco, alcohol, and so on, are abnormal stimulants for insulin secretion. While the body reacts to them by secreting insulin, the response is excessive and therefore harmful to the cells. In addition, the body perceives abnormal stimulants as stress. Even though it reacts by secreting insulin, the body cannot control the damaging effects of the abnormal stimulants. The caffeine, tobacco, alcohol and so on remain in your system, damaging cells.

Ketones

People have confused my nutritional program with a fad diet that requires a drastic reduction in carbohydrates and an equally extreme increase in proteins and fats. This diet causes excessive ketones (a breakdown product of fat metabolism) in the blood that are then excreted in your urine. Advocates of this type of diet give the impression that high-urine ketones are desirable and indicate success. This is not true. Furthermore the diet is extremely dangerous because your body is breaking down healthy tissues and causing imbalances within your system.

Ketones can be used for energy, but when you break down your fat stores too quickly, by extreme dieting, your body cannot utilize the amount of ketones that are released into the bloodstream. That is why excess ketones are excreted in your urine.

Any program that increases the loss of ketones in the urine is also damaging your metabolism at the same time because any extreme form of dieting wastes away lean body mass, as you learned in chapter 2. It is important to note that in all of the diseases where a person wastes away quickly, high levels of ketones are found in the urine.

There is no fast and *healthy* way to lose body fat. Body fat is lost when your metabolism uses your stored fat tissue as energy. If you want to lose body fat you must first heal your metabolism. And as your metabolism heals, it becomes more efficient at burning fat.

The effects of eating excess carbohydrates and man-made carbohydrates are cumulative. So are those that come from stress, dieting, caffeine, alcohol, tobacco, steroids, lack of exercise, stimulant and other recreational drugs, excessive and/or unnecessary thyroid replacement therapy, and all over-the-counter and prescription drugs. If you have been moderate in your eating and lifestyle habits through the years, you may be able to continue moderation and still avoid accelerated metabolic aging.

However, if you are well along on the accelerated metabolic aging track as a result of a lifetime of overindulgence, and if you desire optimum health and longevity, you must do what you can to completely eliminate all destructive behaviors. This may sound impossible and/or overwhelming. And, indeed, eliminating destructive behaviors may be impossible if you are on a program that is, in itself, destructive. The great news is that you will feel immediate benefits from the Schwarzbein Program because it is designed to, first and foremost, *promote good health.* Every day you improve your eating and lifestyle habits you will feel the positive effects. You will sleep better, have more energy, experience fewer cravings and begin to see your body composition changing. Best of all, you will know, by the way you look and feel, that you are reversing the aging process that leads to disease!

Fending off aging and disease is not the only reason to eat a balanced diet. Diet affects mood, which in turn affects behavior. Both mood and behavior seriously impact quality of life on many different levels. Chapter 4 explains how you can regain control over your mood and behavior and, in the process, extend your longevity.

Four

The Low-Serotonin State: The Common Denominator

P atients come to see me with a variety of conditions and complaints. A common denominator with all my patients is that they suffer from a low-serotonin state. Serotonin is a neurotransmitter, one of the chemical communicators in the brain. Neurotransmitters are responsible for communicating the various needs of the body between brain cells and the peripheral cells of the nervous system.

Of course, serotonin is only one of the neurotransmitters that becomes imbalanced through poor eating and lifestyle habits. However, just as we are focusing on insulin as a primary hormone to keep balanced in order to balance all other hormone systems, we will focus on serotonin as a way to balance all neurotransmitters.

Serotonin is one of the major neurotransmitters that affects mood. When serotonin levels are normal, mood is at its best. Normal serotonin levels provide a sense of well-being and contentment. Serotonin is the brain chemical that keeps your focus sharp and your concentration keen, enabling you to get a good night's sleep and to awake happy and energized. When your serotonin levels are normal, you are the most energetic and productive.

When serotonin levels change quickly from high to low, or from low to high, you can experience anxiety, rage, agitation, inability to focus and concentrate, and abrupt sleep disturbances. When levels are at a steady low, you feel depressed, apathetic, lethargic, have decreased memory, lose interest in life and suffer from chronic insomnia. Along with these symptoms you may experience chronic body pain, headaches and irritable bowel syndrome.

A diet sufficient in proteins, fats, nonstarchy vegetables and carbohydrates will provide ongoing serotonin production in the brain. Some of this serotonin is used immediately, and some is stored for future use. But many people, in an attempt to be healthy, have tried very hard to eliminate fat (in turn, cutting protein) from their diet. With very little fat and protein in your diet, your brain will have only enough resources to make a small amount of serotonin, ultimately resulting in a shortage of serotonin—certainly not enough to keep your moods level.

Vanessa's story illustrates how stress, drinking alcohol, smoking cigarettes, using cocaine and eating sugar results in a low-serotonin state, which perpetuates the dependence on stimulants and comfort foods.

Destroying Metabolism Through Stimulant Use

Vanessa: I've always been really thin. I never really thought I looked that great, but I guess I did because in 1980, after college, I got a job on a cruise ship modeling and teaching exercise classes. I was five feet, seven inches and 129 pounds, muscular and strong.

I worked on the cruise ship for five years. On the ship, I ate omelets for breakfast. I didn't drink coffee. For lunch and dinner I'd have a chef's salad or a piece of fish with vegetables and a salad. I don't like desserts so I didn't eat them. It was a very healthy lifestyle, and I loved it.

Then my father was diagnosed with cancer, and I became depressed. I thought a change would do me good. I wanted to learn how to ski and I had friends in Colorado, so I quit working on the cruise ship and moved out there. I got a job at a health club teaching aerobics. I was good at it and entered competitions.

I met and married my husband in Colorado. Before we got married, I thought he was a lot of fun. Little did I know that he had a drinking problem. I became depressed because of my father's cancer and got drawn into my husband's lifestyle without even noticing what was happening. It took three years before my father died. I got more and more depressed as I watched him suffer, wither away and die. Our life was very erratic during that period. My lifestyle gradually changed completely to suit my husband's. He drank bourbon and I drank, too, even though I didn't really enjoy it. For every two or three drinks he had, I would try to drink just one. I drank vodka and orange juice so at least I was getting something "healthy."

Cocaine was part of the party life, too. We did drugs and drank. I would just sip, but when you're doing cocaine all night, a thousand sips makes you a drunk. However, with cocaine you are a very alert drunk. I smoked cigarettes when I drank and did cocaine. I had this craving to keep doing something. When you're buzzed, you need to talk or smoke or drink.

We partied like this four or five nights a week and especially on weekends. Partying changed my eating habits a lot. When you're drinking and doing drugs, you don't want to eat. There were times when I didn't eat all day. When I did eat, I craved sugar. In the morning I felt unhappy, tired and exhausted. I ate doughnuts or cinnamon rolls and drank coffee. I put on fifteen pounds.

Two years after my father died I was in a car accident, which shook me up. I wanted to get away from the party scene and the lifestyle. I told my husband, "You know, I used to be an athletic and healthy person. I would like to get back to that."

We both agreed we needed to change. We decided to move away from the party scene in Boulder to Santa Barbara.

Dr. Schwarzbein: Like Vanessa, many people come to me suffering from depression and addictions, having tried various methods to "cure" their problems. If you binge on carbohydrates or use drugs or other stimulants, understand that the overwhelming desire to use these substances is choreographed by your brain. That is because eating carbohydrates and/or using stimulants raises insulin levels, which results in a rapid release of serotonin from the storage supply in your brain, causing your mood to improve. Of course, when your mood improves, you function better.

While this may seem harmless, it is most definitely not good. Carbohydrates and stimulants cause insulin levels to rise too high, which stimulates an excessive rush of stored serotonin—a *temporary* rush— which is quickly used up. Then, because serotonin levels drop rapidly, you begin to feel down again. This depletion sets up a vicious cycle: You experience the symptoms of low serotonin, and in response you eat an excess of carbohydrates or use stimulants to obtain the rush of serotonin again. You suddenly feel much better. But soon afterward, your mood begins to spiral down again, and your brain demands more carbohydrates or stimulants. This demand for carbohydrates or stimulants is what I call "noise."

When you experience symptoms of low serotonin and have "noise" in your head, it is easy to fall back on overeating carbohydrates or using stimulants to get that rush of serotonin you need to feel better. I always tell my patients not to be hard on themselves. They give in to these cravings not because they are weak but because their brain is telling them that they are not producing enough serotonin. The phenomenon of "noise" in people's heads is a very powerful brain signal that generally cannot be overcome by willpower alone. Everyone reacts differently to the "noise" created by a low-serotonin state. Some people crave "comfort foods," others crave stimulants. The next time you feel the urge to overeat carbohydrates, smoke a cigarette, drink another cup of coffee or have a glass of wine, you now know that it is your brain dictating this strong desire because of low-serotonin levels.

Curing Addictions

The term "addiction" is familiar in our culture. People often speak of conquering their addictions, of "biting the bullet" or going "cold turkey." But curing an addiction does not have to be as grim as that.

As illustrated in Vanessa's story, cravings for all stimulants stem from the same low-serotonin state. The rise in our society of the overconsumption of carbohydrates, recreational drugs, alcohol, caffeine and other stimulants is, in part, due to low-serotonin levels. These are the stimulants that cause an immediate release of serotonin, setting up a vicious cycle of craving that leads to addictions.

Using one stimulant leads to using another. That is because stimulants, whether they are carbohydrates, drugs, alcohol or caffeine, affect serotonin levels in the brain. Caffeine consumption, for instance, causes you to release serotonin, feel pleasurable effects, then experience the drop in serotonin and the subsequent craving for caffeine. This pattern, whether it is caused by caffeine, cocaine, sugar, tobacco or alcohol, is an addiction. Addictions feed on each other. Craving caffeine can cause craving for sugar. Smoking can cause craving for alcohol, and so on. Anyone who has used stimulants understands this craving cycle.

The use of any stimulant will make you dependent on other stimulants to repeat the rush of serotonin. That is why Vanessa felt the desire to smoke, drink alcohol and take drugs, one after the other. This is also the reason why, if you try to quit one addiction, your brain demands that you replace it with another. For example, recovering alcoholics often satisfy their cravings by eating sugar, drinking coffee or smoking cigarettes.

As any addict knows, there comes a time when the stimulant of choice does not produce the desired effect. That is because the storage supply of serotonin in your brain has been used up. No matter how many cigarettes you smoke, cups of coffee you drink, or carbohydrates you eat, you cannot get that rush you so desire. You end up serotonin-depleted, extremely depressed and possibly even suicidal. This is why all stimulants eventually become depressants.

How to Raise Your Serotonin Levels Naturally

In order to halt all cravings and cure depression, you have to make sure you have everything your brain needs to produce serotonin on an ongoing basis. To achieve level moods, you need to eat enough food and good fats to balance insulin and other hormones including estrogen, obtain tryptophan from proteins, and get enough B vitamins, calcium and magnesium from your diet or from supplements. You must also stop the habits that deplete serotonin. When your brain continuously produces enough serotonin so that your mood remains level, your brain will stop demanding substances that will stimulate quick serotonin release from its stores.

To rid your brain of "noise" you must first eat sufficient protein. This is essential because neurotransmitters are derived from dietary proteins. More specifically, serotonin is produced from tryptophan, which is one of the essential amino acids. If you do not eat adequate protein, you will not have enough tryptophan for your brain to produce enough serotonin.

Second, insulin plays a major role in serotonin production by assisting the transfer of tryptophan from the circulatory system into the brain. It is important to note that, while I caution against prolonged high insulin levels, at the same time, serotonin production, which is essential for good emotional and physical health, depends on an adequate level of insulin. The key is balance. Balanced insulin comes from a balanced diet, including adequate fats. When insulin levels are kept too low (by overexercising, not eating enough food or eliminating carbohydrates), you can waste away and may suffer from depression, fatigue, insomnia and osteoporosis.

Estrogen is also one of the hormones necessary for serotonin production. Both men and women have estrogen. Women have much higher levels than men, and these levels change rapidly beginning with perimenopause (the stage in which a woman's peak sex hormone levels begin to drop). Not all women who suffer from low-estrogen states are older women. Younger women who have dieted rigidly, or who have eaten low-fat diets, can also experience low-estrogen states. Men also age and lose peak levels of sex hormones, but later in life than women. Because in men testosterone converts to estrogen, men with low testosterone levels should take testosterone replacement therapy. For those women suffering from low-serotonin symptoms related to low-estrogen states, it is important to find a physician well-versed in *real*[1] hormone replacement therapy. Real hormones are estradiol, progesterone and testosterone, which are identical to the hormones found in the human body, as opposed to drugs like Premarin, Provera and methyltestosterone, chemicals *not* found in the human body.

B vitamins, calcium and magnesium also play an important role in serotonin production. Both vitamin B_6 and magnesium are used up in the body when people take stimulants.

Food Sources of Various Nutrients

B Vitamins: brown rice, chicken, corn, eggs, green leafy vegetables, legumes, meat, nuts, peas, poultry, salmon, shrimp, soybeans, spinach, sunflower seeds, tuna

Calcium: almonds, asparagus, brewer's yeast, broccoli, cabbage, dairy foods, dandelion greens, dulse, filberts, green leafy vegetables, kale, kelp, mustard greens, oats, parsley, salmon (with bones), sardines, seafood, sesame seeds, tofu, turnip greens

Magnesium: almonds, apples, avocados, brewer's yeast, brown rice, cod, flounder, green leafy vegetables, halibut, salmon, sesame seeds, shrimp

Tryptophan: almonds, cottage cheese, peanut butter, peanuts, shellfish, soy foods (tofu, tempeh, etc.), tuna, turkey

---

[1] *Again, because of the misuse of the word "natural" by manufacturers, we use the word "real" when referring to hormone replacement therapy.*

When a patient comes to me with a low-serotonin state, I recommend balanced nutrition and hormone replacement therapy, as needed. I also prescribe: a well-balanced multivitamin; a stress B complex with breakfast; 250 to 300 milligrams of St. John's wort in the morning (slowly increase to 250 to 300 milligrams three times a day, as needed); 1,000 milligrams twice a day of essential fatty acids (capsule or liquid); 250 to 500 milligrams of L-tryptophan(available by prescription only) or 25 to 50 milligrams of 5-hydroxy-tryptophan (5-HTP) (available over-the-counter) at bedtime; and 250 to 500 milligrams of magnesium and 1,000 milligrams of calcium at bedtime.[2]

Essential Fatty Acids		
Omega-3	**Omega-6**	**Gamma-Linolenic Acid**
Flaxseed oil	Canola oil	Black currant oil
Mackerel	Chicken	Bluegreen algae
Salmon	Eggs	Borage oil
Sardines	Flaxseed oil	Evening primrose oil
Tuna	Grape seed oil	
Walnut oil	Safflower oil	
	Sunflower seed oil	
	Turkey	
	Wheat germ oil	

Stress and Serotonin

Another important factor leading to low-serotonin states is emotional stress. Emotional stress depletes serotonin levels without the initial "feel good" release that you get from other stimulants. During times of emotional stress, it is important to make sure that you eat well and take extra care of yourself to replenish your serotonin levels.

---

[2] *If you take too much magnesium you may have loose bowel movements. If this happens, decrease your dose.*

If you do not take care of yourself during this time, you will sink into a chronic low-serotonin state. An emotional trauma can lead to life-long depression and ongoing cravings for stimulants.

Emotional stress brought on by a crisis is not the same as stress brought on by intentionally and regularly putting yourself into high-pressure situations. I have patients who tell me, "I'm addicted to stress," and "I love pressure." The reason these people love stress and pressure is that stressful situations release stress hormones such as adrenaline, cortisol and insulin, which then stimulate the brain to release serotonin. When serotonin is released you suddenly focus better, think more clearly, act quickly and are more productive. This is the "high" that these people are addicted to. When the stress tapers off, serotonin levels drop and so do the good feelings. These people then look for the next pressure situation in order to experience that high again.

Being addicted to stress is also destructive to your health. Stress management is vital to maintaining balanced serotonin levels. Since it takes time to regenerate serotonin, it is important to give your brain a rest from stress. This is accomplished through adequate sleep and stress management.

Addicted to Starvation

Going without food makes some people feel good because they like that "light," "high" feeling they get from an empty stomach and the release of stress hormones, which stimulate the release of serotonin. But stress hormones are limited, so this feeling can be maintained only by using stimulants that mimic stress hormones by releasing serotonin in the brain. This is why chronic dieters often drink coffee and diet sodas and smoke cigarettes—to maintain their serotonin high.

When a person comes to me after years of dieting, I suggest tapering off stimulants to avoid withdrawal symptoms from a rapid drop in serotonin levels. Since people often learn to depend on the good feeling they get from serotonin rushes, an adjustment period occurs. As the person refeeds his or her body with sufficient proteins and fats, he or she will gradually feel better, heal and crave fewer stimulants. This adjustment period reacquaints the body to a steady release of serotonin, and the person finds that he or she consistently feels good.

Even if you are not dieting, you still have to stop stimulants if you want good health and balanced serotonin levels. The good news is that as you eat a balanced diet, take hormone replacement therapy (if needed), and manage the stress in your life, you will have a much easier time quitting addictions. But remember, balancing your serotonin levels is part of healing. And healing takes time.

Stimulants That Initially Release, Then Deplete Serotonin

Alcohol	Ma huang
Amphetamines	Methylphenidate hydro-
Caffeine	chloride (Ritalin)
Carbohydrates (especially	Over-the-counter cold
man-made)	medications
Chocolate	Phentermine (the "phen"
Cocaine and other	in Phen Fen)
"recreational" drugs	Sugar
Dextroamphetamine	Tobacco
sulfate (Dexedrine)	Triiodothyronine (Cytomel,
Diet pills	the active thyroid hormone)

What About Antidepressants?

Another temporary solution to the low serotonin epidemic is to take drugs like Prozac and Zoloft. These drugs are serotonin-reuptake inhibitors, which means they inhibit the disposal of serotonin, thus leading to longer-lasting normal levels of serotonin in the brain. The demands of a low-serotonin society have caused tremendous sales of these drugs in recent years.

However, such drugs are not the panacea. There is no medical diagnosis of a low-Prozac or a low-Zoloft state. The medical diagnosis is a low-serotonin state. Some people feel better when they take these drugs because their serotonin levels are balanced for the first time. This leads them to believe that something is genetically wrong with them. But that is not the case. For most people, a low-serotonin state is not genetic but directly related to eating and lifestyle habits, as well as hormone deficiencies and aging. Taking antidepressants while ignoring the real cause for a low-serotonin state will not yield permanent results. In addition, the side effect of these drugs is that they can cause rapidly changing serotonin levels, which may make you feel worse.

But serotonin-reuptake inhibitors work only if serotonin is available to inhibit. If you suffer from an acute low-serotonin state, even these drugs will not help you. In order for these drugs to work, in the long term you must balance your diet, eliminate the use of stimulants and other drugs, reduce carbohydrate consumption, take hormone replacement therapy (if needed), and manage stress.

Because some patients first improve and then become resistant to the effect of these drugs and some patients do not respond at all, psychiatrists have found that stimulants such as Dexedrine and Cytomel enhance the effects of the serotonin-reuptake inhibitor drugs by increasing the release of serotonin. Though this may not seem bad, these drugs will work only short term. In the same way that the stimulants caffeine, alcohol, stress and sugar deplete your serotonin levels further, so will the stimulants Dexedrine and Cytomel. People are taking two drugs to temporarily correct a condition that is curable by changing eating and lifestyle habits or by taking hormone replacement therapy, if needed.

I am not suggesting that you immediately stop taking your antidepressant drugs, especially if you feel suicidal or extremely depressed. These drugs may save your life. If you are under undue stress, you may need these drugs temporarily, but do not let anyone convince you to stay on them permanently. If you are not currently on these medications, and you are not suicidal, instead of first resorting to drugs to address symptoms, you should do your best to nourish your body so that your brain can make enough serotonin on its own. This cannot be accomplished overnight, but you can reach the goal eventually. Another good alternative is the herb St. John's wort. Start with 250 to 300 milligrams once a day in the morning and slowly increase to 250 to 300 milligrams three times a day, as needed.

Thyroid and the Low-Serotonin State

Because the action of the thyroid hormone is to utilize proteins, to protect against malnourishment your body will decrease thyroid hormone production when you are not eating enough food or are eating an imbalanced diet. If you are given thyroid replacement therapy when your body is in this protective state you will lose lean body mass and become even more insulin resistant.

The symptoms of hypothyroidism and malnutrition are very similar to each other and are often confused: fatigue, constipation, dry skin, cold intolerance, hair loss and weight gain. When patients with these symptoms are misdiagnosed and treated with unnecessary thyroid-hormone replacement[3] (instead of improving nutrition and lifestyle habits), their health continues to deteriorate.

Let me give you a scenario: A woman with poor eating and lifestyle habits (skipping meals, eating a low-fat diet and drinking coffee with

---

[3] Many people who are taking thyroid replacement therapy have asked if they are taking unnecessary or excessive thyroid replacement. You are on unnecessary thyroid replacement medication if you are given thyroid hormone when you do not need it, as in the case above (thyroid blood tests are normal but your symptoms mimic low thyroid). You are taking excessive thyroid replacement if you require thyroid-hormone replacement therapy but are getting too much (this would be determined by a blood test that showed a suppressed TSH level).

artificial sweeteners) goes to her physician with the above-listed symptoms and has blood work done. Her thyroid tests come back in the low-normal range. The doctor fails to ask about her nutrition and lifestyle habits. Without this information, the low-normal thyroid levels are misinterpreted as hypothyroidism instead of malnourishment.

The woman is prescribed thyroid hormone, which *temporarily* alleviates most of the above-listed symptoms: She feels more energetic, her bowel movements become more regular and her weight begins to drop. But again, if she does not improve her eating and lifestyle habits and continues to take thyroid hormone while her body is in this protective state, she will lose lean body mass and become even more insulin resistant.

To make matters worse, thyroid hormone is also recognized in the body as a stimulant because it increases the release of serotonin in the brain. Since all stimulants eventually deplete your body of serotonin, the woman becomes depressed and does not understand why. Obviously she is in worse shape then she was before taking thyroid-hormone therapy.

Next she goes back to her doctor complaining of increasing depression and is prescribed an antidepressant. Again, initially the antidepressant makes her feel better and, ironically, along with the prescribed thyroid hormone (stimulant), the antidepressant is even more effective. Now she is on two drugs, one that releases serotonin from the brain and another that inhibits the disposal of serotonin from the brain. Unfortunately neither of these drugs is working on her problem, malnutrition, which can be cured only by a balanced diet, eliminating stimulants and managing stress.

This woman, who has been given the wrong information, continues thyroid hormones, antidepressants, and bad eating and lifestyle habits, and her health continues to deteriorate. Even though this is a metabolic disaster, the damage can still be reversed by stopping the medicines and addressing her nutrition and lifestyle habits. It is never too late!

Attention Deficit Disorder in Children

Another new fad diagnosis is attention deficit disorder. Attention deficit disorder is due to an imbalance of several neurotransmitters, including a low serotonin level. This diagnosis is on the rise not because we have heightened awareness of it but because more children are becoming serotonin depleted from eating low-fat, high-sugar diets and using stimulants. These children are unfocused and have decreased concentration, mood swings and anxiety. (Teachers often tell me that they notice a drastic change in a child's behavior after that child eats a high-sugar meal.) This disorder is being treated with a combination of stimulants and antidepressants when in fact in many cases it can be corrected only by eliminating stress, sugar and stimulants and providing balanced meals to raise the child's serotonin levels. The best way for children to get proper nutrition from the start is for their parents to eat well themselves. It is very important for the family to eat the same balanced meals while eliminating sugar and other stimulants.

Parents today are extremely concerned about their children's exposure to cigarettes, alcohol and drugs. Keeping your children's serotonin levels balanced is the best guarantee that they will not be tempted by these substances.

Insomnia and the Low-Serotonin State

Insomnia is a major problem in our society. People are taking over-the-counter and prescription sleeping pills or the hormone melatonin instead of addressing why their melatonin levels are low to begin with. However, taking sleeping pills or melatonin is not the solution for insomnia.

The epidemic of insomnia stems from a low-serotonin state. Serotonin is converted to melatonin in the pineal gland in the brain. Melatonin is one of the important hormones that helps you get to sleep and stay asleep all night. When you take over-the-counter melatonin, your own natural production of both melatonin and serotonin decreases, which can lead to more sleep disorders.

Any of the factors that contribute to a low-serotonin state can contribute to a low-melatonin state. You also need cholesterol (found in butter, meat, eggs and shellfish) to make hormones such as cortisol, estrogen and testosterone, which help regulate melatonin production. Also if you do not eat enough food, this will contribute to insomnia by decreasing serotonin production and increasing adrenaline levels.

Serotonin and Longevity

The excess carbohydrates and stimulants you consume to alleviate the symptoms of a low-serotonin state all contribute to chronic high insulin levels. Stress also causes the release of insulin. It is essential to correct all of the behaviors and factors that cause your low-serotonin state in order to keep insulin levels balanced and your mood level. These two conditions are interrelated and essential if you desire overall health and extended longevity.

Again, low-serotonin states are curable. When you understand that the body is interconnected, and that one imbalance creates another, you will understand that balanced nutrition and lifestyle are key to your well-being. Since you are part of the food chain, what you eat and how you live your life creates who you are and how you feel. If you eat properly, manage stress and take hormone replacement if needed, your body can begin to correct your low-serotonin state. Eventually you will find that you no longer crave carbohydrates and no longer suffer from anxiety, agitation, depression, lethargy, poor concentration and lack of interest in life. Symptoms of insomnia, chronic body pain, headaches and irritable bowel syndrome will also be corrected. This will occur so slowly that you might not even recognize it is happening. The only way to recover from a low-serotonin state is to get through the healing process—and it takes time.

Earlier you read that Vanessa was willing and eager to quit using drugs, alcohol, cigarettes, caffeine and sugar. Unfortunately, thinking she was doing the right thing to regain health, Vanessa started a low-fat diet. What she did not know was that her several years of stimulant use and poor eating patterns had moved her well along the road of metabolic aging and insulin resistance. Low-fat dieting then exacerbated all the damage she had already done to her body and delivered a crippling blow to her metabolism.

Gaining One Hundred Pounds in Five Years

Vanessa: That first fifteen pounds I gained when my husband and I were partying didn't upset me. But when we moved to Santa Barbara, I started to have a problem with weight. I stopped drinking, smoking, drugs and coffee so I could get healthy and get pregnant. But I didn't go back to a healthy diet like the one I ate on the cruise ship. I'd wake up every morning and say, "God, I'm fat, I need to lose weight." I started all sorts of different diets, whatever was the rage at the moment. That's when the low-fat thing started to creep in. I started eating a lot more carbs. I was starving all the time. I weighed 158 pounds when I got pregnant with my first child. Then I gained forty more pounds, which put me at 198 pounds by the time my baby was born.

I went back to working out, teaching low-impact aerobics to seniors. I tried to eat well. I lost twenty pounds in the first three months. Then I suddenly stopped losing weight. So I started dieting again.

A year later, I was 180 pounds and still fighting to lose weight. I got pregnant again. I gained another forty pounds. After the baby, I weighed 220 pounds. I went back to work teaching classes, working out and doing everything that I could. Everyone at work said that I needed to go back to the low-fat diet. So I dieted and exercised and couldn't lose weight. Instead, I was gaining. I went up to 229 pounds. I felt so deprived and hungry. I ate low-fat pretzels to replace meals. I don't even like pretzels, but I thought it was "free" food.

I wanted to spend time with the kids before they grew up, so I quit my job. I thought not working at a stressful job and staying on a low-fat diet would help me lose weight. But my weight stayed the same. I didn't have energy. I was hungry and exhausted. My skin was dry. My doctor said that it was because I had two small children. "You are overweight, and you're tired. Lose weight."

I had been a model and had always been the pretty one and was adored for that. Now I was invisible to men. I had never experienced that before. I was so heavy that people I knew didn't even recognize me. I decided that I had to find somebody to help me. That's when my friend said, "This low-fat diet isn't working for you. You need to see Dr. Schwarzbein. She has a diet where you can eat normally and lose weight." I had tried a low-fat diet for five years and gained a hundred pounds. I was ready to try something else.

Dr. Schwarzbein: Vanessa had not only depleted her serotonin levels by using drugs, alcohol, cigarettes, caffeine and sugar; she had also damaged her metabolism by depleting lean body mass. She had developed early insulin resistance.

The Stimulant Trap

People who have destroyed their metabolism (and thus developed early insulin resistance) by using stimulants will always gain weight when they stop using stimulants. This weight gain is generally not caused by overeating but by a metabolic backlash: Stimulants[4] artificially rev up the metabolism by enhancing adrenaline. Among other functions, adrenaline is a protein-utilizing hormone. This means that high levels of adrenaline, or stimulants that enhance adrenaline, will waste away your lean body mass and prevent your body from storing fat in the fat

[4] This stimulant scenario is identical in people who have dieted chronically or who have relied on excessive stress as their stimulant of choice.

cells. At the same time, stimulants decrease appetite so that normal feedback mechanisms for satiety are thrown off, and your brain responds that it is satiated long before your body has met its nutritional requirements. Because stimulants both enhance adrenaline and suppress appetite, the body burns lean mass for energy and becomes protein deficient; as a result you become malnourished.

Furthermore, because you no longer have a fat- and protein-burning stimulant in your system, your true insulin-resistant state emerges: As you learned in chapter 1, there are two vicious cycles of insulin resistance. After years of consuming too much sugar, the cells cannot accept any more sugar molecules, and excess blood sugar is converted to fat and stored in the available fat cells. Also, muscle mass is filled with cells that have insulin-receptor doors to accept sugar. But if you have depleted muscle mass so there are no cells to accept sugar, incoming sugar will be converted to fat and stored in the fat cells. Using stimulants leads to both vicious cycles of insulin resistance.

Subsequent weight gain can be very upsetting to those who have always assumed they were happy and thin because they were "blessed" with a "great" metabolism.

At this point, many people like Vanessa begin to diet thinking they must do something to battle this new weight gain. By going on a low-fat diet, Vanessa destroyed her metabolism further. Low-fat dieting accelerated the damage to her metabolism by *worsening* her insulin resistance, causing her to gain one hundred pounds in five years. I asked her to go on the healing program, which is sufficient in proteins and fats, in order to restore her serotonin levels and heal her metabolism.

Vanessa: I've been on the program for six months. I eat tuna sandwiches with mayonnaise and sprouts and tomatoes, onions, avocados and salad dressings. I feel satisfied and don't need to snack. I lost eight pounds in the first month. I've been exercising and walking, and I'm losing one pound a week. I'm on my way to being the same healthy, athletic woman I have always been.

Dr. Schwarzbein: At this rate, Vanessa could go from 220 to 130 pounds in a year and nine months. Vanessa's story is a good illustration that eating fat does not make you fat. Eating protein and good fats corrects insulin resistance by increasing muscle mass and lowering insulin levels, which means there are more cells and insulin-receptor doors to accept sugar for energy.

Vanessa's story also demonstrates that while stimulants can destroy your metabolism, a low-fat diet accelerates the destruction. If a person indulges in certain high-insulin-producing activities—say, smoking and drinking—but eats well, he or she *might* die at a relatively young age. But if a person is smoking and drinking and eating a low-fat diet, she or he *will* die at a younger age. *Longevity depends on a diet with sufficient proteins and fats to delay insulin resistance for as long as possible, thereby delaying degenerative disease.*

If you exclude fats from your diet, you will increase your risk for all the degenerative diseases of aging. Part II begins with chapter 5, which explains why cholesterol and fat are vital to life.

PART II

Cholesterol and Fat

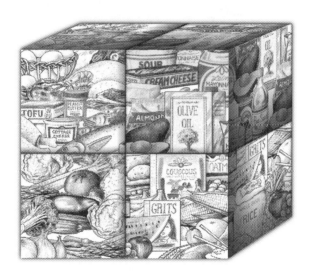

Five

Dietary Cholesterol and Fat Are Essential to Life

The medical profession and the media has so frightened the public about cholesterol and fat that people firmly believe they must be avoided at all costs. For many people today, eggs, butter and red meat represent the fear of cholesterol, and meats, nuts and oils represent the fear of fat. But this fear of cholesterol and fat is not grounded in scientific fact. On the contrary, cholesterol and fat are essential to life. If you do not eat cholesterol and fat, you will be on the accelerated metabolic aging track toward disease and earlier death. What you must understand in order to overcome your fear is that both cholesterol and fat play a major role in what makes you a living being.

Cholesterol and fat are used by the body as building materials for constant replenishment and are supposed to come from dietary sources. Eating cholesterol and fat do not cause heart disease and accelerated death. In fact, you must eat them to avoid heart disease. I have found that the more good fats people eat, the healthier they become.

Cholesterol

Cholesterol is a type of fat that has many functions in the body. Cholesterol is an important structure in cell membranes, keeping the cell membrane permeable so that material can pass easily through the cell. The inside of the cell is also filled with various cholesterol-containing membranes that must be maintained so that the cell can function well.

When your body is comprised of cells that are cholesterol depleted, and thereby less efficient, all the biochemical processes of your metabolism are affected, which means your metabolism cannot function as it should. This overall disruption of efficiency puts you on the accelerated metabolic aging track.

When you deprive your body of cholesterol, an essential building material, membrane structure is altered. When membrane structure is altered, cell growth is disrupted. As a result, there is a potential increase in cancer because cancer arises from abnormal cell division.

In addition, cholesterol is important to maintain normal functioning of various hormone systems and the immune system. Cholesterol is also the structural material from which many important hormones are made, such as vitamin D, dihydroepiandersterone (DHEA), progesterone, testosterone, estradiol, and our major anti-stress hormone, cortisol. Cholesterol is essential for brain function and the stabilization of neurotransmitters. Mood problems such as depression, agitation and irritability can occur when your body does not get sufficient cholesterol.

Cholesterol also forms insulation around the nerves to keep electrical impulses moving. Without this insulation there is an increase in the potential for diseases of the nervous system, such as multiple sclerosis.

Cholesterol can be obtained directly from cholesterol-laden foods, such as butter, meat, eggs and shellfish. You should eat these foods and other types of fats every day.

Functions of Cholesterol in the Body

Essential for brain function

Forms insulation around nerves to keep electrical impulses moving

Forms membranes inside cells

Important structure in cell membranes

Keeps cell membranes permeable

Keeps moods level by stabilizing neurotransmitters

Maintains healthy immune system

Makes important hormones

Fats

One of the problems with convincing people to eat fat is that many people equate dietary fat with body fat. But body fat is only one form of fat, and in fact it is not necessarily derived from the fats that you eat.

Fat is a generic term for structural fats, body fat and dietary fats:

1. *Structural fats* are the class of fats used as building materials within your body for structures such as cells, hormones and brain components.

2. *Body fat* is the reservoir of fat found in fat cells in the form of triglycerides, to be used as insulation and energy.

3. *Dietary fats* come from animal and plant sources. Animal dietary fats are composed of structural fat and body fats. Plant fats are oils that are made up of fatty acids.

When you eat dietary fats, they do not turn into fat on your body because fats do not stimulate insulin release. Fat cannot be stored without the presence of insulin because insulin is necessary to open the doors to store fat in fat cells. No matter how much fat you eat, it does not stimulate the pancreas to secrete insulin. As I have stressed throughout this book, your body is constantly breaking down and building up. Dietary fats play a key role in this replenishing process. Like cholesterol deprivation, fat deprivation disrupts all the biochemical processes of your metabolism, which means that you are on the accelerated metabolic aging track. It would be impossible to list all the health problems that can occur as a result of depriving your body of fat, but here are a few signs and symptoms:

Brittle nails
Carbohydrate and stimulant craving
Constipation
Dry, limp, thinning hair
Infertility
Insomnia
Loss of lean body mass with body-fat gain around the middle
Mood disorders
Scaly, itchy skin

What About Eicosanoids?

When you deprive your body of dietary fats, your body does not get two essential fatty acids: linoleic acid and linolenic acid. Linoleic and linolenic acids are called essential fatty acids because they are required for life; they have to be eaten and cannot be derived in the body. Linoleic and linolenic acid are the building blocks for vital chemicals within the body, including hormones called eicosanoids.

Recently eicosanoids have received a lot of attention in popular literature and are being touted as the most important hormones in the body. However, they are no more important than any other hormone. Every hormone is important for a properly functioning metabolism because all systems of the body are interconnected. Achieving overall balance is the goal.

Balanced eicosanoids are only part of the overall balance you will achieve with proper nutrition. Another way of looking at it is that any imbalance in the body—whether due to a thyroid disorder, menopause, stress or insufficient fat in your diet—will affect eicosanoid production just as it will affect all other hormone production. You should be concerned about the whole system.

Without linoleic and linolenic acid you do not have balanced eicosanoid production; therefore you will experience more allergies, joint pain, reflux, asthma and other conditions and illnesses.

The solution to overcoming these conditions and avoiding many more is to eat good dietary fats. Fats found naturally in nature are healthy. Saturated, monounsaturated and polyunsaturated fats are all natural fats and therefore they are all good for you. (See chapter 25 for more on these fats.)

Your diet should be rich in fat and cholesterol, which should come from a variety of foods such as avocados, butter, eggs, red meat, chicken, shellfish, fish, olives, tofu, nuts and seeds.

Fat and cholesterol are so important to life that your body has backup systems for their production. In fact, one of the most important points this book makes is that the human body can make cholesterol from carbohydrates. Chapter 6 follows carbohydrates through the system to show how they are converted to cholesterol.

Why You Must Eat Cholesterol

By the time patients reach my office, even the most skeptical are ready to hear why eating a low-fat diet is not healthy. Like Robert, Benjamin and Vanessa, anyone who has ever eaten a low-fat diet has suffered the backlash of depriving their bodies of an essential nutrient group. Since there is no better argument than the fatigue, malnutrition, high blood sugar and body-fat gain that they have already endured, my case is made. Of course, everyone wants to be assured that eating cholesterol and fat will not cause heart disease.

The only way to ease people's fears is to begin by explaining how the body is supposed to function on a regular diet of balanced meals.

Your body needs a continuous supply of blood sugar going to your brain at all times. This steady supply of blood sugar is dispersed by your liver. When you eat, the liver prevents excess sugar from reaching the brain. When you are not eating, the liver releases a steady supply of sugar to the brain.

When you eat a balanced meal, the food is slowed by the digestion occurring in the intestinal tract. Over a four-hour period, small amounts of digested food (nutrients) enter the portal vein, which is located between the small intestine and the liver, and pass through to the liver. The liver is a triage station. As nutrients enter your liver, they are sorted so that the liver can regulate how much of the sugar components should pass through. This system works to continually supply your brain and body with sufficient and tightly regulated amounts of blood sugar. Eating balanced meals keeps your body working at its optimum.

However, when you do not eat balanced meals, this process changes significantly. Let's look at what happens when you eat carbohydrates alone.

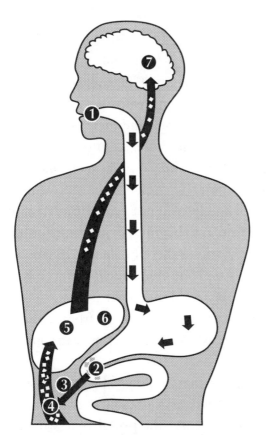

1. You chew and swallow a piece of toast.

2. Bread is broken down into sugar in the small intestine.

3. Sugar leaves the small intestine.

4. Sugar enters the portal vein, triggering the release of insulin.

5. The insulin that is triggered by the sugar alerts the liver and the liver goes into action.

6. In the liver, excess sugar is turned into:
   • Energy
   • Triglycerides
   • Cholesterol
   • Glycogen

7. A tightly regulated amount of sugar is continuously sent to the brain.

Figure 6-1. Following Carbohydrates Through Your System

For example, you eat a piece of dry toast for breakfast. After you chew and swallow that bread it is broken down into sugar in the small intestine. Sugar then leaves the small intestine and enters the portal vein, triggering the release of insulin. (If the blood from the portal vein could be tested, it would show high insulin and sugar levels.) Next, the insulin and sugar go to the liver where insulin communicates to the liver how much sugar has entered.

When you eat excess carbohydrates, the high level of insulin that is released alerts the liver and the liver goes into action. Since the amount of sugar entering the liver is too high to let pass to the brain, the liver must convert some of that sugar into other forms of energy in order to tightly regulate the amount of sugar passing into the bloodstream. The sugar entering the liver can be used as energy or stored as glycogen. If your body does not need energy at the moment or the glycogen stores are full, the liver will convert sugar into cholesterol—which is utilized as building material for hormones, membranes and other structures—and/or triglycerides, which are fatty acids used for energy or fat storage. A tightly regulated amount of sugar continues to be sent to the brain.

It is normal and healthy for insulin to direct the liver to change some sugar into cholesterol and triglycerides. However, this normal process malfunctions when you deprive your body of cholesterol and overeat carbohydrates, or if you engage in any other lifestyle habit that increases insulin secretion.

When you do not eat cholesterol, your body sees this deprivation as a time of "crisis" or "famine." During this "famine," insulin activates an enzyme in your liver called HMG Co-A Reductase that begins to overproduce cholesterol from the carbohydrates you eat. This internal overproduction of cholesterol contributes to the formation of the damaging artery plaque that leads to diseases such as heart attacks and stroke. This is why people like Robert, on low-fat, low-cholesterol, high-carbohydrate diets with high insulin levels, eventually end up with abnormal cholesterol numbers, blocked arteries and bypass surgery.

Consuming excess carbohydrates, while decreasing cholesterol intake, guarantees a steady overproduction of cholesterol within the body.

On the contrary, dietary cholesterol does not play a role in overproducing cholesterol in the liver. In fact, the only "low-cholesterol" diet you can go on is a diet rich in cholesterol. The only way to switch off the enzyme HMG Co-A Reductase is by eating a sufficient amount of dietary cholesterol. Eating dietary cholesterol signals the body that the time of crisis or famine is over. Dietary cholesterol blocks HMG Co-A Reductase. When HMG Co-A Reductase is blocked, cholesterol cannot be formed from sugar. In other words, *the intake of dietary cholesterol stops the internal production of cholesterol.*

I have heard people say, "If my body can make its own cholesterol, why do I have to eat it? I'll stay on my low-fat diet and let my body make all the cholesterol it needs." But this strategy will not work. Carbohydrates stimulate insulin, and all the processes leading to plaqueing of the arteries are caused by the overproduction of insulin. Equally important is that carbohydrates do not have the same ability as dietary cholesterol to signal the body when it has made enough cholesterol. So the body keeps producing more cholesterol. When you restrict dietary cholesterol and force the body to make its own cholesterol, your body makes more cholesterol than it needs. For example, when you eat a meal that contains cholesterol, such as a breakfast of eggs with toast and butter, your body does not need to make any extra cholesterol. But if you eat a meal that does not contain cholesterol, such as a breakfast of cereal with skim milk, fruit and orange juice, your body overproduces cholesterol from these foods. And when you have too much cholesterol derived from high insulin levels, you are more likely to develop coronary artery plaqueing and subsequent heart disease.

Drug companies are well aware of the function of the enzyme HMG Co-A Reductase. This knowledge has led to the invention of drugs that switch off production of cholesterol in the body by blocking HMG Co-A Reductase. These are the so-called "Statin" drugs.

Drug companies continue to market these drugs while researching new drugs to switch off cholesterol production in the body, instead of simply telling people to eat cholesterol and decrease sugar and stimulant consumption. Eating cholesterol is the only healthy way to block cholesterol production in the body. Eating cholesterol is one of the best things you can do for your body.

It is important to emphasize that insulin is the major hormone directing the overproduction of cholesterol in the body. Regardless of what causes insulin to rise, the body responds to elevated insulin levels by overproducing cholesterol. High insulin levels are caused by stress, dieting, caffeine, alcohol, aspartame, tobacco, steroids, lack of exercise, stimulant and other recreational drugs, excessive and/or unnecessary thyroid replacement therapy, all over-the-counter and prescription drugs, and eating a diet insufficient in proteins and fats while eating excess carbohydrates.

Part III examines three formidable degenerative diseases of our age: heart disease, Type II diabetes and cancer. Beginning with chapter 7, you will learn why heart disease is not caused by high cholesterol levels in the blood system but by the high-insulin lifestyle habits that lead to these abnormal cholesterol profiles.

PART III

Heart Disease, Type II Diabetes and Cancer

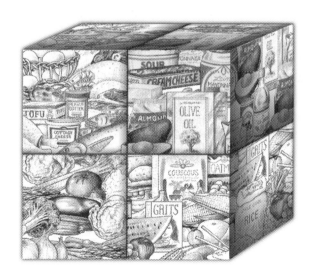

Seven

Your Cholesterol Count Is Not the Final Word

J oel, a fifty-five-year-old man, had a history of high cholesterol levels and was very confused about what he should or could do to improve his cholesterol profile. Specifically, Joel was concerned about his total cholesterol number because he was told that if he could lower his total cholesterol number, he could decrease his risk for a heart attack.

What Are Lipoproteins?

Total cholesterol numbers are derived by adding together the three different cholesterol-carrying proteins known as lipoproteins (*lipo* = fat): high-density lipoproteins (HDLs), low-density lipoproteins (LDLs) and very low-density lipoproteins (VLDLs). Cholesterol and triglycerides (fats) are water insoluble, but packaged into these water-soluble proteins they float freely through the bloodstream, which is mostly water, hence the name lipoproteins.

Your lab cholesterol-profile report shows the results of the triglycerides, total cholesterol, HDL, LDL and VLDL levels. These levels are all mathematically related to each other in the following ways: Total cholesterol = HDL + LDL + VLDL; (VLDLs = triglycerides divided by 5. Therefore triglyceride levels contribute to your total cholesterol level. Another way of putting it is that total cholesterol = HDL + LDL + triglycerides divided by 5.) HDLs are proportional to one over the VLDLs (HDL $\propto$ 1/VLDL). In other words, the higher one level the lower the other level, and vice versa. This means that if your HDL levels are high, your VLDL levels will be proportionally lower.

As you can see, the total cholesterol number is only a mathematical equation, the sum of all the cholesterol carried in the three major lipoproteins: HDLs, LDLs and VLDLs. Since HDLs, LDLs and VLDLs all perform different functions in your body, adding them up to arrive at a total cholesterol number does not tell you anything. In other words, there is no such thing as a "normal" or "abnormal" total cholesterol number. Furthermore, you can have a heart attack with what everyone calls "normal" total cholesterol numbers; conversely, you can end up living a long life with what people call "abnormal" total cholesterol numbers.

Joel was a perfect example of someone who focused on one number and did not view his health as a total picture. He had been eating a low-fat diet to lower his total cholesterol number, but instead his total cholesterol number had gone much higher. This led him to believe that his abnormal cholesterol problem was genetic and there was nothing he could do about it. But Joel had come to the wrong conclusion. There was a lot he could do to improve his health.

Joel: Before cholesterol was ever an issue, I was concerned with diet because I was one of these kids who had terrible acne. Back in the 1950s, they felt that diet influenced acne. "No chocolate" were buzzwords. No fatty products, no dairy products. I remember doctors saying to me, "You don't have to have dairy. You don't need calcium—you're an adult."

So I got that advice but my diet growing up was typical American. Candy bars? Yeah sure. All the time. Dessert? You bet. Never had a clue that *sugar* was a problem.

Back then nobody cared about cholesterol levels either. The first time I can remember being aware of high cholesterol numbers was in my twenties when I went in for a life insurance policy. I came back to my doctor and said, "How come you didn't say that I had a problem? The insurance company wants to charge me more for being a high-risk case."

He said, "It's not that big a deal and you're almost within normal." My total cholesterol number, I believe, was somewhere between 260 and 270.

Since the first time I learned my cholesterol numbers were high, I've wanted to find the right diet to reduce my cholesterol. Then I heard that fat is bad for you. At that point, I was beginning to put on a little weight and, thinking fat's bad for you in terms of increasing weight gain and cholesterol, I cut out the fat.

Every time somebody came along and said you should do this or not do that, I listened. So I created my own crazy diet and had some do's and don'ts that I exercised over many, many years.

I kept trying to do the healthy thing. Every morning I got up and drank a huge glass of fresh orange juice. Then I had huge bowl of cereal with skim milk. What American doesn't think cereal is good for you? If I really wanted to be extra healthy, I put berries or other good fruits on my cereal. I'd have a cup of coffee, too. Around lunchtime I'd crash. Because I wanted to stay thin, I'd have fruit juice for lunch, and by mid-afternoon I had no energy again. I was having to come home and take a nap almost every afternoon for an hour or two. Later in the day I'd come home and immediately feel so down in the dumps I'd have two, three or four cocktails, which once again shot me up.

During that time, my cholesterol numbers kept getting worse. I received the most ominous report of all when I applied for more life insurance. My numbers were the highest they ever were, in spite of the fact that my diet was, in my opinion, better than ever. I had gotten used to it. I thought, this is my unique genetic makeup as a human being. My metabolism. This is me. There's not a thing that can be done about it. So here I was, fifty-five years old and still in the dark.

Then my wife, who had a twenty-eight-year history of migraine headaches, heard about Dr. Schwarzbein. She made an appointment and, per Dr. Schwarzbein's instructions, catalogued her diet over a two-week period prior to the visit. I went along to try and fill in the blanks of her case history. We told my wife's story.

Dr. Schwarzbein put my wife on estrogen replacement therapy. Then she said, "Aside from taking estrogen, we are going to change your diet." She began to explain her theories on nutrition. I was mesmerized.

Dr. Schwarzbein didn't have a clue as to why I was all excited and asking questions. At one point, she said to my wife, "Now I'm going to have you see our nutritionist to get you on a program that is going to make you healthier."

I said, "How about me?"

She said, "What's your problem?"

"Well, for one thing, high cholesterol."

"What do you eat?

"Gee, a big bowl of blah, blah, blah." I was bragging about my low-cholesterol diet. I said, "I don't know why I have a problem." I told her about my lunch of fruit juice. I told her about the alcohol and then collapsing.

She said, "I'm going to put you on a program that will help all of that. We can start to change your cholesterol metabolism in a week or two."

Dr. Schwarzbein: Joel remembers when the medical community first looked at fat and cholesterol as being the cause of heart attacks. By the early 1960s, medical science became interested in preventing heart attacks after researchers came to the conclusion that butter had the same chemical constituency as the measured cholesterol in the blood and the waxy buildup in arteries. Because researchers wanted to understand how they could alter this process, studies were launched to find out which lifestyle habits contributed to heart attacks. Unfortunately, too many variables were either left out or missed. Instead of illuminating the causes of heart disease, these studies actually contributed to the vilifying of dietary cholesterol.

Why Do We Focus on Cholesterol Numbers?

Like Joel, most people over the last thirty years have come to believe that reducing or eliminating cholesterol from their diets will decrease their risk of heart attacks. This is not so. *The only way to prevent a heart attack is to evaluate your entire lifestyle, and then take appropriate steps to improve it.* But people have a very hard time believing this, given the information they have received from their physicians, the media and drug manufacturers. Ironically, "Effect of Diet and Smoking Intervention on the Incidence of Coronary Artery Disease," the landmark study that launched the fear of cholesterol (appearing in the December 12, 1981, issue of the medical periodical *Lancet*) actually proves what I tell my patients about cholesterol, lifestyle and heart attacks. I will walk you through this study, the results and the outcome.

In Oslo, Norway, researchers tracked a group of 1,232 men considered to have a higher risk for coronary heart disease because they smoked and had high total cholesterol levels. The men were split into two groups: an intervention group and a control group. Members of the control group were told to continue their lifestyle as they had in the past. The men in the control group were given a checkup once a year, but they were not given any guidance or suggestions regarding their lifestyle.

The intervention group was given much more attention. In the intervention group, those with high triglyceride levels were given specific instructions to stop smoking, eat less sugar, drink less alcohol and reduce cholesterol intake. Every six months, researchers encouraged them in their efforts to improve their eating and lifestyle habits and reduce smoking and drinking. At the end of a five-year period, the intervention group had decreased their heart disease and death by 47 percent over the control group. Their triglycerides had dropped by 20 percent compared to the control group's. Their total cholesterol levels had dropped 13 percent lower than the control group's.

Unfortunately, this study was misinterpreted, with tragic results. The intervention group had been able to cut back their smoking by an average of 45 percent compared to the control group. But it was not recognized at the time that smoking altered cholesterol numbers. Even though researchers analyzed the decreased tobacco consumption as possibly playing a role in the decreased risk for heart disease, they discarded the evidence. The success of the study was attributed to eating less cholesterol instead of to smoking fewer cigarettes. Researchers concluded that decreasing cholesterol intake was the *sole* reason for the great success of the intervention group. This conclusion made an enormous impression on the medical community, and the low-fat movement was launched.

In fact, however, the Oslo study did *not* demonstrate that reducing dietary cholesterol was the cause for the 47 percent reduction in risk of heart attack and death. The men in the intervention group showed that decreasing smoking lowers insulin levels and, subsequently, cholesterol and triglyceride levels. The reason is that anything that lowers your insulin levels will cause you to reap all the benefits of a healthier lifestyle, including reducing your risk for heart disease.

But because the results were misinterpreted, people like Joel were told to focus solely on achieving a lower total cholesterol number by eliminating cholesterol and fat from their diet. And if low was good, lower must be better.

People have been taught that their total cholesterol numbers will provide an assessment of their *risk* of a heart attack. But your total cholesterol number is not a good predictor of *having* or *dying* of a heart attack. Statistically, there are just as many people having and dying of heart attacks with total cholesterol levels below 200 as there are with total cholesterol levels above 200.

I understood that getting Joel's focus off his total cholesterol number was not going to happen in the first visit. So instead I directed him to look at his stress, his alcohol and caffeine consumption, and his low-fat, low-cholesterol, high-carbohydrate diet. I felt it would be more productive to focus on eliminating obviously harmful behaviors than it would be to start off talking about the numbers he was so worried about. Joel and his wife both sat with my nutritionist and learned more about the healing program.

> **Joel:** It was like Woody Allen's movie *Sleeper.* It was like somebody coming down to Earth and saying, "Oh yeah, eggs, they're good for you— eat them every day. Skim milk? Nah—use real cream." What was bad one day became good the next. What was good that day became bad the next.
>
> Dr. Schwarzbein's nutritionist, Robin, suggested we do our shopping on the periphery of the supermarket. Wow, what a powerful visualization. On the periphery are all your fresh things. Real food. And yet two-thirds of the market is clogged up in the middle with all the junk. Robin gave us guidelines on what to eat and what not to eat. We began the program instantly and with gusto. We went out to lunch to a place that she recommended, and we were laughing like kids because we were eating all these things we were previously not supposed to eat. I said, "Whoa, this is exciting—this is terrific. But I don't believe for one second I'm gonna get my numbers down."

> **Dr. Schwarzbein:** It was not Joel's total cholesterol number that was dooming him to an early death. It was his high-insulin lifestyle—stress, alcohol and caffeine consumption and a low-fat, low-cholesterol, high-carbohydrate diet.
>
> I explained to Joel that reducing his cholesterol intake was not the way to reduce his risk of a heart attack. You can achieve the "perfect" cholesterol profile by going on a low-fat diet and/or using cholesterol-lowering drugs and still die of heart disease. This is because high total cholesterol numbers are not the cause of heart attacks. A high-insulin lifestyle is the cause of heart disease.

Insulin and Heart Disease

All of the processes leading to plaqueing of the arteries are caused by the overproduction of insulin. We know this from studies on insulin and clogged arteries (plaqueing) that started in the 1960s. In the most startling study, "Effect of Intraarterial Insulin on Tissue Cholesterol and Fatty Acids in Alloxan-Diabetic Dogs," published in 1961 in *Circulation Research*, researchers actually infused insulin into the femoral arteries of dogs. Plaqueing of the arteries occurred in every dog, demonstrating that insulin causes this to occur.

Stress, dieting, caffeine, alcohol, aspartame, tobacco, steroids, lack of exercise, stimulant and other recreational drugs, excessive and/or unnecessary thyroid replacement therapy, all over-the-counter and prescription drugs and, most important, eating a diet that is insufficient in proteins and fats while eating excess carbohydrates, will increase your insulin levels. This will lead to early insulin resistance and heart disease.

Life Is More Than a Number

Like Joel, we all tend to focus on numbers. We focus on cholesterol numbers, blood pressure numbers, chronological age and the number on the bathroom scale. But the fact is this: If all you ever do is try to bring your numbers down as low as possible, you will generate chronic health problems and disease. This is evident if you read the case histories in this book. Robert almost died from malnutrition while trying to bring his cholesterol numbers down. At the same time he suffered two heart attacks, in addition to irritable bowel syndrome and reflux. Elizabeth and Vickie, whom you will read about later on, focused on the number on the bathroom scale and suffered from Stein-Leventhal syndrome, premature osteoporosis, anorexia and bulimia and depression. Joel ate a low-fat diet because he believed he was doomed to have a heart attack, but he actually increased his risk for heart disease while suffering from fatigue, weight gain, anxiety and depression.

Just as I encourage people to avoid looking at the number on the bathroom scale, it is even more important that people stop looking at their cholesterol numbers as the deciding factor in assessing their health, or as the determining factor in whether or not they will develop heart disease.

> Because systems of the body are interconnected, good health is related to more than one thing. We have to remember that, when we look at a cholesterol profile, it is simply one tool for assessing a person's health. An "abnormal" cholesterol profile would be only one marker indicating the health of your metabolism. Likewise, a "normal" cholesterol profile does not indicate that you are not at risk for heart disease. Instead of looking at a number, ask yourself questions about your lifestyle. Are you living a healthy life, or are you stressed, eating poorly, using stimulants and other drugs, and not exercising?

Joel: P.S., the dietary program did work. I started exercising. One thing leads to the next. If you're not feeling good, you can't exercise. And if you're not exercising you don't feel good. I've been feeling better and living better, and there is no doubt in the world that it's due to the lifestyle changes I've made.

I went on this program to feel better and I lost fifteen pounds without trying. I cut out booze for three months completely. Now I'm back to moderation.

If you're on a mission to increase your total cholesterol count, be fatigued and depressed, I was on the diet to do that. This low-fat, high-carb rigmarole is calculated to make you feel lousy, squash your immune system, maybe make you malnourished and, in the final analysis, wind up with big total cholesterol numbers.

Dr. Schwarzbein: The fact that Joel's cholesterol panel did improve is incidental compared to all the other positive eating and lifestyle changes he was able to make. Like Joel, you should focus on maintaining a healthy lifestyle that will result in balanced insulin levels. Different cholesterol numbers will emerge as you balance your eating and lifestyle habits. Some people will have a total cholesterol below 200 to match their healthy lifestyle, and some people will have one above 200 to match *their* healthy lifestyle. Balanced nutrition and lifestyle are vital to well-being—what you eat and how you live your life determine who you are and how you feel. *Ignore your cholesterol numbers and focus on your total lifestyle and you will likely live a long and healthy life.*

You may argue that, while total cholesterol is not the definitive number, there are still reasons to look at your cholesterol profile—like noting the risk ratios, for example. If you are still not convinced, chapter 8 will further explain why you should not focus solely on your cholesterol profile any more than you should focus solely on your total cholesterol number.

Eight

What About the Good HDLs?

L ike Joel, one of my patients, Miriam, worried that her abnormal cholesterol profile would lead to a heart attack. Her father had died at a relatively young age of a heart attack. Her concerns focused on a history of low HDLs because she was told that HDL is the cholesterol lipoprotein that should be high. When she came to me, she had been trying to raise her HDLs by following a low-fat, vegetarian diet.

Miriam: After my father's first heart attack, I began watching my diet by eating chicken and low-fat cheeses and other low-fat foods. I ate oatmeal for breakfast instead of eggs. Everyone was saying, "Don't eat eggs."

My father died of a massive heart attack in 1982 at age sixty-eight. I was thirty-six. My dad's death freaked me out because we have the same genes. At the time, Pritikin was saying, "Don't eat oils. Don't eat fat." I disciplined myself and said, "Okay, I'm going to continue to do the Pritikin diet."

I went in for my first cholesterol reading when I was forty-one and it wasn't really too bad. My HDLs were around fifty, but I thought it would be nice to have them a lot higher than that. The total cholesterol reading was something like 136. At the time everyone thought, oh that's great, it's wonderful to have low total cholesterol numbers. Even my doctor thought that. However, he wanted my HDLs to be a lot higher. He didn't make a big thing out of it other than mentioning that there is fat in chicken, and so on. So I stopped eating chicken and started pretty much being a vegetarian. I ate mainly legumes, rice, pasta, grains, vegetables, beans and some fish. Later on I got more eccentric about it and gave up fish, too.

I had my cholesterol checked regularly and my HDLs were going down, down and down, clear into the thirties. I became so fearful of my cholesterol problem that I quit having it checked. I felt my fear and anxiety around my HDL levels were only making matters worse.

By 1995 I was eating mostly carbohydrates, thinking I was getting enough protein from legumes.

When I was forty-nine, I was really anxious and out of sorts. I was still having a menstrual period so other doctors said I was fine. You know, most doctors won't give you hormone replacement therapy until you've missed periods for a year. They'll give you tranquilizers, though. I didn't want to do that so I went on living with the anxiety for a few months until a friend said, "You've got to see Diana Schwarzbein." And that was it.

I went to see her in October 1995. I was a nervous wreck about my HDLs, menopause and everything. She put me through her entire checkup. I said, "Don't tell me what my HDLs are." They wrote on my chart, "Do not tell patient the reading." I only wanted to know when it got better. I didn't want to know how bad it was.

Dr. Schwarzbein: Miriam, like Joel, feared dietary cholesterol as the sole cause of heart disease. But this fear is unfounded in science. As you learned in chapter 6, dietary cholesterol does not cause heart disease.

I explained to Miriam that it was important for her to eat fat in order for her to reduce her risk for heart disease. Eating saturated fats like butter increases the proportion of HDLs in the bloodstream. (HDL lipoproteins are considered good because they take cholesterol back to the liver and therefore are thought to protect against heart disease by keeping your arteries clean.)

Her current diet, which was low in fat and high in carbohydrates, was depleting her estrogen levels, and the body needs good estrogen levels to raise HDL levels. Ironically, her diet was also causing high insulin levels, which could eventually lead to plaqueing of the coronary arteries!

I explained that she did not want to totally eliminate cholesterol from her bloodstream because cholesterol is essential for life. I advised her to begin eating foods containing healthy fats and cholesterol. I also prescribed sex hormone replacement therapy.

Miriam: Dr. Schwarzbein told me about the diet to raise my HDLs. I changed completely overnight. Even though I was skeptical, what she told me made sense, and I trusted her.

Dr. Schwarzbein said you need olive oil. You need flaxseed oil. You need canola oil. You need butter. You need to eat nuts that are high in fat.

I'm such a perfectionist. I was trying to do everything perfect and change overnight. My family thought I was a complete basket case because here I was preaching no fats, and all of a sudden I was telling them to eat eggs. They thought I was crazy. My sister said, "Are you sure you know what you are doing?"

I said, "I'm not sure of anything, but I'm going to eat eggs because what Dr. Schwarzbein told me made sense."

I'm trying to make the right improvements to my diet. I'm eating a lot of soy products, salmon, almonds and peanuts—foods I had been avoiding.

Dr. Schwarzbein: In addition to having a fear of saturated fats, patients like Miriam have told me that they avoid eating meat or animal products because they contain added hormones.

It is true that much of our food is adulterated. Whenever possible buy hormone-free, antibiotic-free, range-fed meat and poultry. On the other hand, the benefits you get from eating meat and animal products are that these foods supply your body with the needed resources to fight off chemical additives or hormones. In other words, depriving your body of those needed resources leaves you without defenses. In a culture where it is difficult, if not impossible, to get unadulterated food, being left without defenses is very dangerous.

Miriam: I had an HDL reading of 55. Really a great increase. I'm a perfectionist so it would be great to get it up in the sixties or seventies, but we will see.

Dr. Schwarzbein: Even though Miriam would like to see her HDL number go up to 60 or 70, her ideal number may be 55. Again, she should be more concerned about her lifestyle, not any single number. It was her eating and lifestyle habits that determined her risk for heart disease, not her HDL number. She should not focus on her total cholesterol number nor should she focus on her cholesterol risk ratios. Cholesterol profiles are only one indicator of the potential risk for a heart attack.

You could eat too many carbohydrates, drink alcohol, smoke tobacco, ingest artificial sweeteners, eat damaged fats[1], drink caffeinated beverages or be too stressed, and your cholesterol panel could look perfectly normal for the time being. But these bad habits destroy your body on a cellular level, and this destruction cannot be detected immediately by a blood test. In the meantime, while your blood tests look normal, your body is making cholesterol and triglycerides at a very high rate, because all of these lifestyle habits raise insulin levels. Remember that the liver converts sugar into fats when insulin levels are elevated. Your body can then store or use these fats for energy; therefore, the blood levels do not immediately change.

Abnormal cholesterol panels are a *late* indicator of abnormal cholesterol metabolism. The damage being done on a cellular level from overconsumption of carbohydrates or use of stimulants has to occur for years before an abnormality will show up on a blood panel. That is true even if the damage is substantial.

The following two examples show hypothetical ideals of HDL, LDL and VLDL lipoproteins.

---

[1] *Damaged fats, which are trans-fatty acids, oxidized and hydrogenated fats, are covered extensively in chapter 26.*

Example One: Which cholesterol panel do you think is better?
Panel 1: Total cholesterol 240 = HDL 80 + LDL 140 + VLDL 20
Panel 2: Total cholesterol 240 = HDL 40 + LDL 170 + VLDL 30

When evaluating the three lipoproteins, higher HDLs and lower VLDLs are desirable. By following a healthy lifestyle, HDLs increase and VLDLs decrease. So Panel 1 is much better than Panel 2. But note that the sum of the lipoproteins of each panel both arrive at the same total of 240. Hence total cholesterol levels are meaningless.

Example Two: Which cholesterol panel do you think is better?
Panel 1: Total cholesterol 240 = HDL 60 + LDL 160 + VLDL 20;
      Tg = 100
Panel 2: Total cholesterol 180 = HDL 60 + LDL 80 + VLDL 40;
      Tg = 200

In comparing these two cholesterol panels, you want the VLDLs and the triglycerides to be lower even if this means accepting higher total cholesterol and LDL levels. Therefore Panel 1 is the better panel.

The last example illustrates why cholesterol panels do not show your risk for heart disease. Furthermore, it demonstrates how easy it is to misinterpret cholesterol profiles.

Example Three: This example is from two different people. Which one has the lower risk for a heart attack?
Person 1: Total cholesterol 180 = HDL 60 + LDL 100 + VLDL 20
Person 2: Total cholesterol 180 = HDL 60 + LDL 100 + VLDL 20

Without knowing anything about these people's eating and lifestyle habits, there is no way to determine their individual risks or which one of them has the higher risk of a heart attack. Their doctors would likely tell both of them that they were low risk. But you now know that the risk of heart attack has nothing to do with cholesterol numbers but everything to do with where you are on the accelerated metabolic aging track, which is dictated by eating and lifestyle habits.

This may make sense to you. On the other hand, you may have also seen that decreasing your fat intake, combined with exercise, improved your cholesterol numbers. So now you are confused.

Do Exercise and Eating a Low-Fat Diet Reduce the Risk for Heart Disease?

Low-fat advocates have encouraged a very dangerous trend in this country. People are going on rigorous exercise programs and low-fat diets to improve their cholesterol profiles and to decrease their risk for heart attacks. But the truth is, more people are dying of heart disease by eating a low-fat diet, with or without exercising.

Still, many people are convinced that eating a low-fat diet and exercising is the way to reduce heart attacks. That is because in the beginning of the low-fat movement, people combined low-fat eating with exercise and saw the good results in their cholesterol profiles: lower VLDLs, LDLs and higher HDLs. (Remember: if your VLDLs are lowered, your HDLs will rise proportionately.) Of course after seeing these initial results, their commitment to the low-fat diet was reinforced.

However, those same people eventually saw those great results reversed. Some thought that it was because they were not exercising enough, and exercised more. Others thought they needed to cut even more fat from their diet, and they did. Others still, including many members of the medical community, did not know how to explain what had happened. So they blamed genetics: "Your father died of a heart attack so you probably will too." Unfortunately, this fatalistic argument was convincing and many people accepted their poor health as genetic, putting up with illness and decreased quality of life. But genetics is not the issue here.

You can see *initial* good results with a low-fat diet. When you exercise and eat a low-fat, high-carbohydrate diet, excess carbohydrates will be turned into cholesterol and fats that are then used by the body as energy. During this stage, your cholesterol profile will significantly improve. But a low-fat, high-carbohydrate diet burns muscle mass, especially if you are exercising. This causes your metabolism to slow down, which in turn *lowers* your requirement for energy. Now any excess carbohydrates you eat will be converted into cholesterol and not used. Over time, your cholesterol levels will rise.

As I said earlier, when people finally reach my office, they are eager to hear the truth about low-fat diets. I explained to Miriam that exercise combined with balanced nutrition is the way to lower her risk for a heart attack. If she ate fat and cholesterol and focused on improving her lifestyle, she would live a longer and healthier life. Because Miriam is a perfectionist, she wanted to know exactly how to improve her lifestyle and all about the real risk factors for heart disease.

Chapter 9 will explain the real risk factors for a heart attack.

Nine

The *Real* Risk Factors for a Heart Attack

Through the media we hear that longevity is increasing and that deaths from heart attacks are decreasing. It seems reassuring. But it is not as promising as it sounds. It is true that *death* from heart attack is going down. But the *incidence of heart attack* is going up and is appearing in individuals ten to fifteen years younger than it did twenty years ago.

More people are also living longer with heart disease. You can now call 911 and have paramedics arrive quickly on the scene to save your life. This means you can have a heart attack and not die within the first twenty-four hours. But just because we have been able to keep patients alive after a heart attack does not mean that we are suffering fewer heart attacks. Regardless of how it is presented, the rise in heart attacks is a fact, and the total amount of people with heart disease is increasing. Even with all the new forms of medical intervention—including cholesterol-lowering drugs and bypass surgery—heart attacks are still the primary cause of death in this country and in all other industrialized nations.

The Two Types of Heart Attacks

Atherosclerosis, or plaqueing of the coronary arteries, leads to heart attacks. There are two forms of atherosclerosis. One is a solid continuous wall of plaque and the other is a liquid core of cholesterol plaque. Let me explain how these two types of plaque buildup differ, and lead to different types of heart attacks.

We used to see mostly the type of heart attack that occurred from a slow buildup of a solid continuous wall of plaque as a person ages. When the buildup of plaque formed a column from one side of the artery to the other, almost totally blocking blood flow, a person became symptomatic. For example, he or she might experience chest pain during exercise. This is known as angina. Even if a person does not experience angina, this wall of plaque was easily detected by treadmill tests and angiograms. Through symptoms or testing, a person could be informed of his risk. At that point medical/surgical intervention could prevent a heart attack. However, not all intervention works 100 percent of the time; so if the blockage continued, or if a clot formed in the remaining blood-flow space, a heart attack could still occur.

Heart attacks caused by the process of plaque buildup used to occur at a much older age. As explained above, these heart attacks were almost always preceded by the warning symptoms described. Now higher numbers of relatively young people are having heart attacks without experiencing any chest pain—even when they may have recently had a perfectly normal treadmill test or angiogram.

The reason is that this type of asymptomatic heart attack results from a different type of plaque buildup. Instead of a solid buildup of plaque that forms like a column on the artery wall, a lesion with a liquid core of cholesterol forms. This liquid core is directly related to excess sugar being converted into cholesterol inside arterial cells, and is exacerbated by any habits that raise insulin levels. Since this lesion does not completely block the artery wall, it is possible for a lesion to form without producing any symptoms or being detected by the standard diagnostic tools (treadmills and angiograms). Since a person does not know he or she is at higher risk, no steps are taken to prevent a heart attack.

Over time the cholesterol liquid core continues to grow, and the pressure increases inside it. Eventually, the lesion erupts and the liquid core solidifies in the bloodstream, totally blocking blood flow and producing a heart attack.

I have had patients say, "My internist told me not to worry. I will never have a heart attack with *my* cholesterol numbers!" Unfortunately, the risk for heart attack can never be completely eliminated, and it is possible to have either type of heart attack at any age—you cannot eliminate normal aging processes, and a heart attack is a part of the normal aging process. On the other hand, you *can* eliminate your risk for the type of heart attack resulting from liquid-core cholesterol plaqueing by improving your eating and lifestyle habits, which will reverse accelerated metabolic aging.

Risk Factors for Heart Disease

Abnormal cholesterol metabolism—Related to lifestyle

Age—Older than fifty-five years

Gender—Male greater risk than female

Genetics—6 to 10 percent attributed to genetics

High blood pressure—Related to high insulin and arterial wall damage

High insulin levels—Directs biochemical processes that lead to plaqueing

Menopausal status—Low estrogen promotes clotting

Midsection body-fat gain—"Insulin meter" indicates insulin resistance

Sedentary lifestyle—A factor in insulin resistance

Stimulants—Cause hormone imbalances that promote clotting, cellular growth and inflammation

Stress—Causes insulin resistance

Tobacco—Causes insulin resistance

Type II diabetes—End-stage insulin resistance

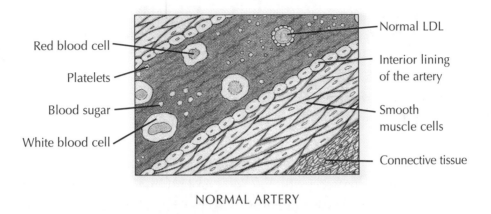

Red blood cell

Platelets

Blood sugar

White blood cell

Normal LDL

Interior lining of the artery

Smooth muscle cells

Connective tissue

NORMAL ARTERY

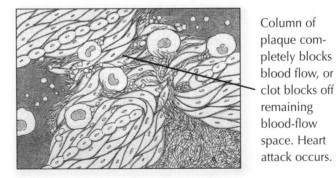

Slow, continuous clogging in the artery, forming a column of plaque

PARTIALLY BLOCKED ARTERY

Column of plaque completely blocks blood flow, or clot blocks off remaining blood-flow space. Heart attack occurs.

COMPLETELY BLOCKED ARTERY

Figure 9-1. The Solid, Continuous Wall of Plaque

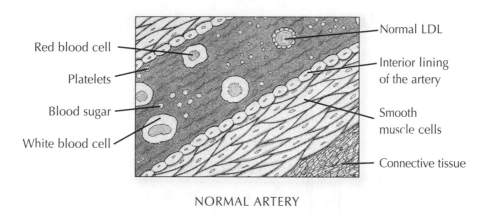

Red blood cell

Platelets

Blood sugar

White blood cell

Normal LDL

Interior lining
of the artery

Smooth
muscle cells

Connective tissue

NORMAL ARTERY

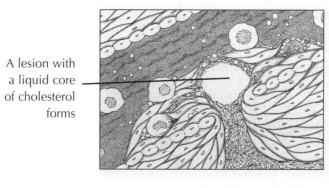

A lesion with
a liquid core
of cholesterol
forms

ARTERY WITH LESION

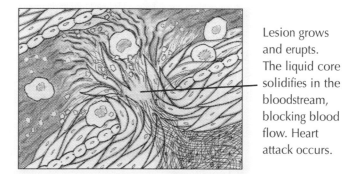

Lesion grows
and erupts.
The liquid core
solidifies in the
bloodstream,
blocking blood
flow. Heart
attack occurs.

ARTERY WITH LESION ERUPTING

Figure 9-2. The Liquid Core of Cholesterol Plaque

Risk Factors for Heart Disease

Abnormal cholesterol metabolism: Abnormal cholesterol metabolism can lead to abnormal cholesterol profiles. Abnormal cholesterol profiles are only one risk factor for heart disease. Abnormal cholesterol profiles indicate that you have had prolonged elevated insulin levels. Prolonged elevated insulin levels lead to heart disease. Again, you can have "normal" cholesterol numbers and still have increased insulin levels. Therefore a normal cholesterol profile by itself does not indicate a decreased risk for heart disease.

Age: The older you get, the more chance you have of developing heart disease. This is because you become more insulin resistant with age. As your cells age, they do not process sugar as well. And if your cells are not using sugar for energy, your body, directed by insulin, will turn that excess energy into cholesterol. Chronological age is always a factor in heart disease. However, if you have been on the accelerated metabolic aging track through bad eating and lifestyle habits, you can have a heart attack at a much younger age.

Gender: Men have a higher risk of heart disease than women because men have higher levels of testosterone, which lead to overall lower levels of HDL. One of the reasons testosterone increases the risk for heart attack is that testosterone increases insulin secretion, leading to increased tendency to clot, increased blood pressure and earlier insulin resistance. On the other hand, estrogen thins the blood and keeps arteries flexible, which means that women have a lower risk for heart disease than men.

Genetics: Researchers confuse genetics with lifestyle habits. But as you learned in previous chapters, degenerative diseases have little to do with genetics but mostly are acquired through poor eating and lifestyle habits. In fact, "The Nurses' Health Study: Twenty-Year Contribution to the Understanding of Health Among Women," published in the 1997 issue of the *Journal of Women's Health*, clearly states that, ". . . the contribution of genetics to most major chronic diseases remains small. For breast cancer, for example, perhaps 6 to 10 percent can be attributed to inherited genetic factors. A similar estimate may prevail for colon cancer and for heart disease. Thus, the study of lifestyle factors acting in the broader population is more useful in identifying areas for prevention in the general population than merely focusing on the high-risk sub-groups for specific diseases."

The minor role that genetics plays in heart disease risk may be attributed to the fact that some people secrete more insulin and other hormones in response to various stimuli. This can lead to metabolic aging in a shorter amount of time if the person engages in high-insulin eating and lifestyle habits.

High blood pressure or hypertension: People with higher blood pressure have higher rates of heart disease. High blood pressure is defined as the top number (systolic) blood pressure greater than or equal to 160, and the bottom number (diastolic) blood pressure as greater than or equal to 90. These readings have to be observed on at least three different occasions before a diagnosis of high blood pressure is established. The causes of sustained elevated blood pressure are high blood volume and stiff artery walls.

Think of your arteries as tubes that cannot expand significantly when overfilled. As the volume of fluid passing through them increases, the pressure exerted on the walls of the tube also increases. The more pressure in the arteries, the more damage to the wall of the arteries. It is in these high-pressure areas that arterial plaqueing begins.

High insulin levels result in high blood pressure in two ways:

1. Insulin causes an abnormal increase of salt retention at the kidney level. Increased salt in the system increases water retention. More overall fluid means higher blood pressure.

2. Insulin overstimulates the nervous system, which increases blood pressure. The amount of blood pumped out by each contraction of the heart is increased, and the artery wall becomes stiffer.

High insulin levels: In 1996, *The New England Journal of Medicine* published a paper: "Hyperinsulinemia as an Independent Risk Factor for Ischemic Heart Disease." This paper concluded that, "high fasting insulin concentrations appear to be an independent predictor of ischemic heart disease in men." If you are interested in reading this or more studies on this subject, they are listed in the References section at the end of this book.

Menopausal status: Doctors generally tell menopausal women to go on a low-fat diet to prevent heart disease. However, the first course of action in a case where menopause could be a risk factor should be estrogen replacement therapy. Women who do not take estrogen replacement therapy have a much higher rate of heart attacks than women who do take estrogen. Hormone replacement therapy slows down the accelerated metabolic aging process by improving insulin resistance, which keeps cells younger. Estrogen also thins the blood and keeps arteries flexible. Replacing estrogen decreases the risk of heart disease for every woman.

Low sex hormones in men are not as common. Men with low DHEA and low testosterone levels have a higher risk for heart attacks than men with normal hormone levels. These hormones are metabolic markers of aging. Low DHEA and testosterone levels in men younger than fifty-five indicate accelerated metabolic aging. The cause of this type of low DHEA and testosterone levels is, in part, due to poor eating and lifestyle habits. The first course of action is to improve your habits, not take hormones. If you do take hormones, you should still address eating and lifestyle habits and be monitored closely by a physician who is well-versed in real hormones. Ironically, cholesterol-lowering drugs lower DHEA and testosterone levels.

Midsection body-fat gain: This is the "apple shape" body configuration. Your midsection is where you first notice fat deposits from prolonged high insulin levels. Your midsection is your "insulin meter." This also applies to people who may not be excessively overweight but are soft around the middle.

Sedentary lifestyle: Being sedentary contributes to heart attacks because overall insulin levels are higher when you are sedentary. Exercise lowers insulin levels; therefore regular exercise has been linked to a lower incidence of heart attacks.

Stimulants: Stimulants cause insulin resistance, lead to abnormal cholesterol production, and increase heart rate and blood pressure. Stimulants also raise stress hormones, which cause increased inflammatory responses, cellular growth and blood clotting—the three primary factors in plaque formation.

Stress: Stress triggers the "fight-or-flight" response by first releasing the stress hormones adrenaline and cortisol. In prehistoric humans, this response was intended to mobilize sugar stores for quick muscle action and quick thinking. When sugar starts to rise in the bloodstream, insulin is released. This rise in insulin serves two distinct purposes. The first is to get the increased sugar into the cells, the second is to counterbalance the rise in sugar so that you do not get high blood-sugar levels that would be harmful to the brain.

Stress also increases the level of other stress hormones (eicosanoids). These hormones are responsible for normal blood clotting, but when elevated they can produce clots that lead to heart attack. That is why many heart attacks occur during periods of great stress.

The fight-or-flight response is a good short-term reflex when you need to act quickly. However, constant stress causes prolonged elevated insulin levels, leading to plaqueing of the arteries.

Tobacco: Smokers have a higher risk for heart disease. Nicotine in tobacco stimulates the release of insulin, leading to insulin resistance. Medical studies have recently confirmed that smokers have an increased risk of developing Type II diabetes. Type II diabetics have the highest risk of heart disease. Tobacco smoke oxidizes cholesterol by both introducing and increasing the generation of cholesterol by both introducing and increasing the generation of free radicals within your body. Both damaged cholesterol and increased free-radical production increase the rate of arterial plaque formation.

Type II diabetes: Type II diabetics have the highest risk of heart disease because of prolonged high insulin levels. Type II diabetes is the end stage of insulin resistance, and heart disease is the leading cause of death in these patients.

Keeping your arteries free of plaque is primary in avoiding a heart attack. This can be achieved through balanced eating and lifestyle habits. Balanced eating means eating sufficient proteins, fats, non-starchy vegetables and carbohydrates according to your current metabolism and activity level. Balanced lifestyle habits include stress management, adequate exercise, good sleep habits, avoiding drugs, stimulants and artificial chemicals.

Eating excess carbohydrates is one way to raise insulin levels and thereby develop insulin resistance and degenerative diseases. The story of Riley, in chapter 10, illustrates how smoking is another habit that eventually results in insulin resistance and Type II diabetes.

Ten

Two Packs of Cigarettes a Day x Fifty Years = Accelerated Metabolic Aging

E veryone knows that cigarettes increase the risk for lung cancer and chronic lung diseases such as emphysema. But cigarettes also destroy you at the cellular level and can lead to Type II diabetes, as in the case of Riley.

Riley Milligan is a seventy-three-year-old man I have treated for four years for Type II diabetes. Riley and his wife Melba came to see me on the advice of Melba's daughter, Sandra. Riley's stepdaughter was concerned about Riley's foot lesion, which would not heal.

> **Melba:** My husband, Mr. Milligan, was a truck driver, and in 1978, when he was fifty-five years old, he got a physical to renew his license. At that time, they told him he was a borderline diabetic. Three months later he found out he had a full-blown case of diabetes. He saw a doctor and was put on some kind of oral medication.
>
> In 1992, we moved to California to live. He had this sore spot on the top of his foot which would not heal, and that's when we went to Dr. Schwarzbein.
>
> At that time, his blood sugar was over 300, his cholesterol and everything was high. The first thing she said when she looked at his medicine

was, "We're throwing this stuff away. This is not good for diabetes, and it isn't helping you one bit." She talked to us about the diet she wanted him to go on. As soon as we heard about it, I looked at him and he looked at me, and I thought, *This is impossible; it will never work because my husband loves to eat.* Everything that he shouldn't eat is what he liked better than anything else. He loved hamburgers, french fries, spaghetti, Mexican food, doughnuts, cakes, pies, mashed potatoes with gravy. I thought, *There's no way this will ever work.* I never thought he would do it.

Dr. Schwarzbein explained everything. We saw the dietitian that day and a physical therapist for exercise. They put him on an exercise program. He had a lot of trouble with his feet and legs and could not walk far at all. He would just give out. At that time his weight was 205 pounds, and he's five feet, seven inches. He was way overweight. Dr. Schwarzbein's own words were, "He was a total mess."

We left with a diet he could start on, and in two weeks we had to go back.

Dr. Schwarzbein: I explained to Riley and Melba that "borderline diabetes" did not really mean anything. By the time someone is diagnosed with high blood-sugar levels, she or he has been on the accelerated metabolic aging track for a very long time. Type II diabetes is a metabolic continuum involving both insulin and sugar levels. A healthy person starts off with normal insulin and blood-sugar levels. High-insulin eating and lifestyle habits cause insulin resistance. Insulin resistance is characterized by high insulin levels and normal blood-sugar levels. If a person continues high-insulin eating and lifestyle habits, insulin resistance will worsen. The next stage is both high insulin and high blood-sugar levels. This is Type II diabetes.

At one time, Riley had been a heavy smoker. The hydrocarbons in tobacco damage cells directly, and damaged cells have fewer insulin cell doors. The nicotine in tobacco stimulates the release of insulin, and overexposure to insulin also results in fewer cell doors. Also, nicotine enhances the hormone adrenaline which causes the breakdown of lean body mass. A decreased response of cells to insulin's actions is termed "insulin resistance." (See chapter 1 for more on insulin resistance.) Medical studies have recently confirmed that smokers have an increased risk of developing Type II diabetes. Type II diabetes is a sign that you have been on the accelerated metabolic aging track for a very long time.

Though there was one other known diabetic in Riley's family—his newly diagnosed ninety-five-year-old mother—Riley's diabetes was not hereditary. His diabetes was caused by his two-pack-a-day cigarette habit which spanned fifty years, along with his high-starch diet.

Riley's stepdaughter, Sandra, was wise to be concerned about Riley's foot lesion. Poor wound healing is associated in diabetics with high blood sugars and can lead to amputations. One reason for this is that the white blood cells of the immune system that help to heal wounds are too sluggish when blood sugars are elevated. Consequently they do not move well to the area of injury. Also, high blood sugars feed the wound with sugar, which delays the healing process.

Smoking was also the cause for his legs "giving out on him" when he walked. This is called claudication; the arteries feeding his legs were blocked and when he exercised his feet ached. This is analogous to anginal chest pain. When you have a blocked artery in your heart and you exercise, you experience pain because you are not getting enough oxygen to your heart. Likewise, when you have a blocked artery in your legs, you experience pain when you exercise because not enough oxygen is getting to your legs. However, metabolism is resilient, so Riley definitely benefited by quitting smoking a year earlier.

But, in addition to the wound and his other symptoms, Riley was overweight and terribly out of shape. I was very concerned about him.

Despite being on a high dose of oral medicine to lower blood-sugar levels, Riley had initial blood sugars near 300. We stopped his oral diabetes drug because, to lower blood-sugar levels, it raises insulin levels. Since Type II diabetes results from overexposure to high levels of insulin over time, I did not want to continue a medication that would push his insulin higher. I knew that a treatment program combining regular exercise, a cutback in stimulants and other drugs, and a diet lower in carbohydrates would reduce Riley's insulin and blood-sugar levels. No pill in the world can accomplish that.

I asked Riley to test his blood sugar before and one hour after meals. With that information we would be able to evaluate his numbers and make changes in the number of carbohydrates he could have per meal. The goal was to keep his one-hour, post-meal blood sugars at less than or equal to 160. (Nondiabetics never get this number above 140, even if they eat sweets.) He was also instructed to try some form of physical activity but not overdo it.

I asked Riley to see me every four weeks that first year. I wanted to monitor him and encourage him. An older person has a harder time breaking bad habits, and Riley was a starch lover who had no exercise program.

Melba: The first couple of weeks were terrible. It was just as though he was not getting anything to eat. He was used to eating anything and everything he wanted and any amount he wanted. It was just hard for him to change that.

But Riley was so determined to help himself that he ate frequently, but just a very small amount of what was on the diet. At the end of two weeks there was a little improvement. Dr. Schwarzbein explained everything again. We were going in there every four weeks the first year. He started improving slowly. He started losing body fat. His diet was very strict. Very low carbohydrates. But that's what started working. I made him "Anytime Soup," which was just chicken, carrots, onions and tomatoes [see recipe, page 331]. He could have that soup anytime. Carbohydrates were cut to fifteen grams per day.[1] That's really nothing. Then at the end of a month, she allowed him to have forty-five grams. The next month, she put him up to sixty grams. In three months, he was up to one hundred.

The weight was just coming off of him. He went from a forty-two-inch pant down to a thirty-six within a year. Now his weight stays between 171 and 174 pounds. His diet is very flexible. There are many, many foods he can eat. I learned how to prepare foods with very little carbohydrates that taste very good.

---

[1] *Because Type II diabetics have high blood-sugar levels, they can reduce carbohydrate consumption this low. The reason is that diabetics can use their already-high levels of blood sugar in lieu of eating carbohydrates. But once their blood-sugar levels normalize, they, too, cannot maintain a drastic low-carbohydrate diet. I recommend that Type II diabetics* not *reduce their carbohydrates this low unless they are being closely supervised by their physician. Furthermore, drastically reducing carbohydrate consumption (less than forty-five grams per day) is extremely dangerous for a nondiabetic.*

Riley: I feel fine about the diet now. Once in a while I'll get the sugar craving and I'll eat a little bit of it. It will drive my blood sugar a little higher, but usually it will come right back down. I feel good. My health has improved 100 percent.

Dr. Schwarzbein: With his strict adherence to the nutritional program and his progressive exercise regimen, Riley brought his blood sugars under control in no time. He lost body fat and his wound healed.

Riley's metabolism was ruined by a fifty-year cigarette habit, no exercise and a carbohydrate-rich diet that accelerated his aging process. But even after fifty years of doing the wrong things, Riley began to reverse the metabolic aging process by balancing his own insulin levels through nutrition and lifestyle. Riley is an example of someone improving the worst possible metabolism.

Along with heart disease and Type II diabetes, the incidence of cancer has also dramatically increased over the past twenty years. People come to me because they want to get healthy and they know that I am committed to preventive medicine. A very common question is, "How can I prevent cancer?" Of course, I cannot give a definitive answer, but I can explain the obvious risks. Chapter 11 will explore the risks for cancer.

Eleven

Cancer and the High-Insulin Lifestyle

C ancer is a general term for diseases that are characterized by uncontrolled, abnormal growth of cells that is caused by damage to cellular DNA. Cancer develops in one tissue and can then metastasize (spread) through the bloodstream and lymphatic system to other parts of the body.

Cancer, as well as being the second-leading killer (behind heart disease) in today's statistics, is still on the rise. The types of cancer most dramatically rising over the past twenty years are breast, prostate and colon cancers. The dramatic increase in these cancers has paralleled the growth of the low-fat movement. Here is how that probably happened: Early studies linked these three cancers to excessive body fat. Those studies were improperly interpreted to conclude that eating fat made you fat and also caused cancer. So people cut more fat out of their diet and replaced it with carbohydrates. This helped propel the popularity of the low-fat movement. And we continue to hear that cancer is on the rise because people are not cutting enough fat from their diets. But this argument does not make sense. If eating a low-fat diet prevents cancer, then why do people on low-fat diets—those who are thin as well as those who are overweight—continue to get cancer, and at an even higher rate?

If you look at those early studies, the real risk factor is evident. While authorities acknowledged that excessive body fat was a risk factor for cancer, they did not recognize the *cause* of this risk factor. The real reason that excessive body fat is linked to cancer is that elevated insulin levels cause excessive body fat, rapid cell growth and an imbalance in every other hormone system of the body. When hormones are imbalanced, the possibility of abnormal cell division increases.

Instead of advising people to eat good fats and cut down on excess carbohydrates, ingested chemicals and stimulants, the medical professionals told people to do exactly the opposite: Eat a low-fat, high-carbohydrate diet. People consumed less and less fat while increasing consumption of artificial foods and stimulants. Since fats are essential for hormone production, which regulates normal cell division and keeps immune systems functioning, avoiding fats left people defenseless against cancer-cell growth. The low-fat movement was a big mistake, and the dietary advice it popularized has caused the alarming rise in cancers that paralleled this advice.

Cancer risk increases with aging. Anything you do to age your body faster, thereby accelerating the metabolic aging process, increases your risk for cancer. Anything you do to elevate the levels of growth hormones will lead to increased risk/growth of cancer. Likewise, anything you do to lower the levels of growth hormones to normal levels slows down metabolic aging and decreases the risk of cancer.

Factors That Increase the Level of Growth Hormones and Damage Cellular DNA

Diet
A low-fat diet
Aspartame
Certain natural stimulants, such as ma huang
Excess carbohydrates and/or sugar

Factors That Increase the Level of Growth Hormones and Damage Cellular DNA (continued)

Drugs/Chemicals	Lifestyle Habits
All prescription and over-the-counter drugs	Alcohol
Exposure to, or ingesting, chemicals	Caffeine
Steroids	Skipping meals
Unnecessary and/or excessive thyroid	Stress
hormone	Tobacco

Factors That Lower the Level of Growth Hormones

Reversing the above bad habits
Exercise
Good oils and fats
Good fiber
Hormone replacement therapy, if needed
Stress management

Since aging will always remain the number-one risk factor for cancer, we will never be able to definitively prevent cancer. However, we *can* address the obvious risk factors for accelerated metabolic aging through eating and lifestyle changes.

Increased Risk Factors for Cancer

Age: Normal aging plus bad eating and lifestyle habits damages cellular DNA

Cholesterol-lowering drugs: Very low cholesterol levels increase abnormal cell division

Eating "damaged" fats: Causes damage to cellular DNA

Eating excess carbohydrates: Increases insulin levels and other growth hormones

Environmental exposure to toxins: Damages cellular DNA

Increased Risk Factors for Cancer (continued)

Genetics: Some genes predispose you to different types of cancer (this applies to only less than 10 percent of all cancers)

Ingesting stimulants: Affect the body the same as stress

Insulin: Increases the growth-factor insulin out of normal range

Stress: Immune-system function declines under stress. Stress stimulates secretion of various growth hormones.

• • • •

Age: Physiologically, the aged have one thing in common: Their cells are metabolically old. Cellular DNA is more likely to have become damaged over the years, which can lead to uncontrolled abnormal replication of cells. Cancers arise from such abnormal cell division and growth.

Cells, under the direction of hormones, are constantly replicating and dividing in order to keep up the ongoing replenishment process within the body. As we age, hormone levels decline, and this imbalance can lead to abnormal cell division.

Another reason the elderly are at higher risk for cancer is that the immune system declines with age. The immune system is a surveillance system for the body; it watches not just for foreign substances like viruses and bacteria but also for cancers.

Elderly people have many years behind them. Those who have enjoyed good eating and lifestyle habits throughout their lives will not be as prone to degenerative diseases as those who have indulged in bad habits. But the effects of *any* bad eating and lifestyle habits are cumulative. The results of those cumulative bad habits are manifested in advanced aging of the immune and hormone systems. In other words, your age is relative to where you are on the accelerated metabolic aging track. If you are on the accelerated metabolic aging track due to high-insulin eating and lifestyle habits, both your immune and hormone systems will have aged faster. And prolonged high insulin levels are one of the causes of the accelerated metabolic aging process, which is responsible for rising cancer rates among the aged and, increasingly, among younger individuals.

Cholesterol-lowering drugs: Cholesterol-lowering drugs have been implicated in increasing cancer risk. In January 1996, in the *Journal of the American Medical Association,* a Special Communication article, "Carcinogenicity of Lipid-Lowering Drugs," was published with the following conclusions: "Patients to whom these drugs are prescribed, either singly or in combination, are exposed throughout many years to doses approaching those shown to be carcinogenic in animals." Since cholesterol is an essential constituent for cell membranes, trying to lower the amount of cholesterol in the body leads to decreased cholesterol for normal cell-membrane division. When there is not enough cholesterol for normal cell membranes, abnormal cell division and abnormal growth can occur, both of which increase the risk of cancer.

Cholesterol is used in the body to make hormones, so without cholesterol you have abnormal hormone production, which leads to abnormal cell division.

Eating damaged fats: Eating damaged fats damages cellular DNA, resulting in accelerated metabolic aging, which leads to cancer. (See chapter 26 for more on damaged fats.)

Eating excess carbohydrates: Again and again in this book, I have emphasized that high carbohydrate consumption will put you on the accelerated metabolic aging track. Eating an excess of carbohydrates will damage your metabolism. Eating an excess of carbohydrates can cause cancer by increasing insulin levels and other potent growth hormones while at the same time damaging cellular DNA faster because excess sugar is an oxidant. Not eating enough carbohydrates is as bad as eating too many. When insulin levels are kept too low, the body breaks down more than it builds up.

Environmental exposure to toxins: Exposure to environmental toxins—such as radiation, chemical fumes, household and industrial solvents, pesticides, insecticides and other poisons, ultraviolet rays, exhaust, smog, and so on—damages cellular DNA. Damaged cells are more likely to divide abnormally.

Genetics: It is irrefutably known that there are genes that, when "turned on," lead to various cancers. However, this still remains one of the lowest risk factors for cancer in the general population because most DNA mistakes are acquired, not genetic. (This applies to only less than 10 percent of all cancers.)

Ingesting stimulants: Your body reacts to stimulants exactly the same way it does to stress. Stress and stimulants both affect the same hormone systems that lead to prolonged elevated insulin levels and accelerated metabolic aging.

Insulin: Hormones play an important role in normal cellular replication. Hormones are growth factors that cause cells to replicate. Normal cell division and growth are regulated by numerous growth factors in the body. If growth factors become imbalanced, cancer may occur.

A potent growth factor is the hormone insulin. In tumors, it has been found to accelerate growth and division. Breast, colon and prostate cancers have been found to grow more rapidly under the stimulus of insulin. Anything you do to increase the growth factor insulin beyond normal range will increase your risk for cancer. Thus, eating and lifestyle habits that lead to prolonged high insulin levels will increase your risk of cancer.

Stress: Stress stimulates secretion of various growth hormones, including insulin. Immune system function declines under stress. People tend to eat more comfort foods (cookies, doughnuts, ice cream) when stressed because stress causes serotonin levels to drop. Rapid decreases in serotonin levels lead to carbohydrate craving and other stimulant craving. Need for alcohol, caffeine, sugar and tobacco intake goes up under stress. Lifestyle habits deteriorate. People tend to exercise less because the stressful situation is consuming their relaxation time. There is truth in the old axiom, "Stress kills."

Many patients have told me that they believe that saturated fats cause cancer. But, to the contrary (as you read in chapter 8), saturated fats promote health. If eating fat gives you cancer, then the French, the Inuit and the Tibetans—to name a few high-fat cultures—would have higher rates of cancer than we do. But they actually have lower rates of cancer than we do. What they have in common is that they all eat a lot of good, healthy fats, which do not damage cellular DNA, as do damaged fats.

It is common sense that anything people do to improve their overall health should lower their risk for developing cancer. Remember that fats are an essential nutrient group and are part of a healthy regimen; they are essential for sustaining hormones, normal cell division and a healthy immune system.

Scientists and researchers are constantly looking for the cause of cancer. Popular literature frequently speculates on diets or lifestyle changes that can prevent cancer. But cancers are not caused by any one factor. All lifestyle factors contribute either to good health or bad health. Studies proving that insulin is a growth factor for breast cancer are available in the medical literature. Understanding that insulin is a growth factor in cancer should be enough to convince people that eating and lifestyle habits that cause prolonged high insulin levels will put them at increased risk for cancer.

As we know, cancer arises from uncontrolled cellular division due to DNA damage and prolonged high insulin levels. The older we are, the more likely this can happen. Any of the factors that cause the accelerated metabolic aging process will contribute to cancer. Of course, once cancer is diagnosed you need to listen to the expert medical opinions and choose a course of treatment that you are comfortable with. I am not against surgery, chemotherapy or radiation for the treatment of cancer. (However, I would like to see an all-out emphasis on cancer prevention.) But once the cancer-fighting measures have been implemented, we should focus on rebuilding and rebalancing the normal tissues left. These normal tissues have also been affected by the chemotherapy or radiation therapy, and they need proper care as the body recovers from this traumatic process. Proper care would include balancing nutrition during and after treatment, in addition to balancing hormones, getting sufficient exercise, avoiding all toxins (including sugar, caffeine, alcohol and tobacco) and eliminating stress as much as possible. Knowing the risks of cancer will help you make educated choices.

Most people want to take responsibility for their lives and do the right thing to attain balance and promote their own health. Part IV will clarify how you can achieve balance by eating from all four nutrient groups and by consuming carbohydrates according to your current metabolism and activity level. Chapter 12 begins by answering: "What is a carbohydrate?"

PART IV

Achieving a Balanced Diet

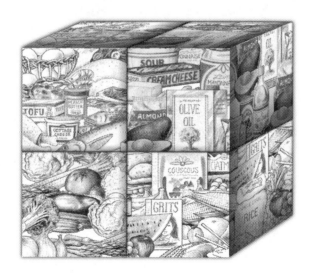

Twelve

Carbohydrates
Are Sugar

C arbohydrates are chains of sugar molecules. Carbohydrates are
either simple or complex. Simple carbohydrates are defined as
one to two connected sugar molecules. Complex carbohydrates are three or more connected sugar molecules. Carbohydrates
are found in both real and man-made foods such as whole grains,
starchy vegetables, fruits, most dairy products, breads and cereals,
pasta, and sweets. Both complex carbohydrates (vegetables/grains)
and simple carbohydrates (fruits/candy) are broken down in the
digestive track to one-sugar molecules. Therefore, all carbohydrates
are sugars.

Insulin and Glucagon

How your body utilizes the carbohydrates (sugar) you eat is determined by the ratio of insulin to glucagon—the two main hormones
produced in the pancreas to regulate nutrient distribution.

Glucagon is an important hormone for mobilizing nutrients.
Glucagon directs the liver to release sugar, which raises the levels of
blood sugar available for the brain and body. Glucagon also directs

cells to release fat that can be used as energy and to release proteins that can be used as building materials.

Insulin is the most important hormone for nutrient storage. Insulin is responsible for putting nutrients (proteins, fats and sugar) into cells. This process of unloading sugar and other nutrients from the bloodstream into cells is vital for two reasons. As nutrients are put into the cells, the body is replenished and refueled, and blood-sugar levels are balanced, protecting the brain. Also, insulin tells the liver that too much sugar has entered, and the liver reacts by increasing fat production from that incoming sugar.

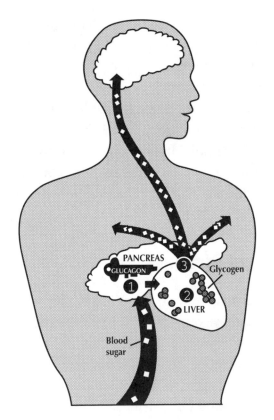

1. Low blood-sugar levels signal the release of glucagon by the pancreas.

2. Glucagon stimulates the liver to break down glycogen stores into blood-sugar molecules, which enter the bloodstream.

3. Tightly regulated amounts of sugar pass through the liver to the brain and body.

Figure 12-1. How Glucagon Works

The ratio between these two hormones determines whether food will be used as building materials or fuel, or stored as fat. A low ratio (a higher proportion of glucagon) means that more food will be used as building materials or fuel. A high ratio (a higher proportion of insulin) means that more food will be stored as fat.

Glucagon is released in response to protein foods. Insulin is released in response to carbohydrates and some amino acids. Neither is released when nonstarchy vegetables and fats are consumed. Therefore, if carbohydrates are eaten alone, the insulin-to-glucagon ratio is too high. If proteins are eaten alone, the insulin-to-glucagon ratio is too low. If fats

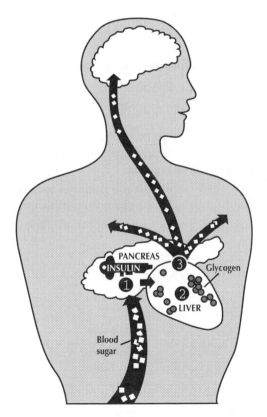

1. High blood-sugar levels signal the release of insulin from the pancreas.

2. Insulin stimulates the liver to convert sugar into energy, glycogen, triglycerides or cholesterol.

3. Tightly regulated amounts of sugar pass through the liver to the brain and body.

Figure 12-2. How Insulin Works

The Net Effect of the Insulin-to-Glucagon Ratio Over Time

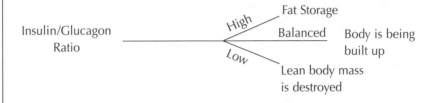

Insulin/Glucagon
Ratio

High
Low

Fat Storage

Balanced   Body is being
built up

Lean body mass
is destroyed

Glycemic Index of Foods

❶ When you eat a processed carbohydrate such as white bread:

Refined carbohydrates are rapidly digested into sugar, which is quickly absorbed into the portal vein, causing a rapid rise in insulin.

❷ When you eat a complex carbohydrate such as whole wheat bread:

Complex carbohydrates are digested at a slower rate so that less sugar arrives at the portal vein all at once. Less insulin is secreted in response, but it is still above a balanced level.

❸ When you eat a balanced meal such as chicken, baked potato with butter and a nonstarchy vegetable such as broccoli:

Digestion is slowed down even further when you eat a balanced meal of proteins, fats, nonstarchy vegetables and carbohydrates. This results in a balanced level of insulin, which remains level for a longer period of time.

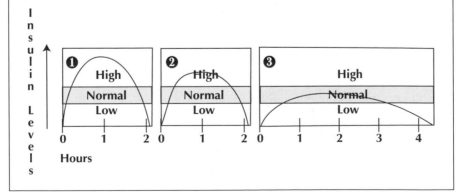

Insulin Levels

❶ High
Normal
Low

❷ High
Normal
Low

❸ High
Normal
Low

0   1   2   0   1   2   0   1   2   3   4

Hours

or nonstarchy vegetables are eaten alone, there is no effect on the insulin-to-glucagon ratio. If you eat a mixed meal of proteins, fats, nonstarchy vegetables and carbohydrates, you will have a balanced insulin-to-glucagon ratio, which is the goal.

The Glycemic Index of Foods

In addition to the above, the insulin-to-glucagon ratio is also determined by the glycemic index of foods: a measure of how fast insulin rises in response to the amount of sugar entering the portal vein at any given moment. The faster sugar arrives, and the higher the amount of sugar entering the portal vein, the higher the glycemic index of that food. In general, simple sugars arrive faster than complex sugars; therefore, simple sugars have a higher glycemic index than complex carbohydrates.

Whole grains have a lower glycemic index than their refined counterparts. The fiber in the whole grain slows the rate of absorption of sugar into the system, lowering the insulin-to-glucagon ratio. But the refining process removes this protective coating of fiber, as in white rice.

Why Balanced Meals Are Important

More important is how you combine the four nutrient groups. For example, if you eat only a potato for dinner, the glycemic index of that meal is higher than if you ate that potato with salmon, broccoli and a salad. This is why: Carbohydrates enter the bloodstream much faster than proteins and fats do. Carbohydrates cause insulin release, but they do not cause glucagon levels to go up. When you eat excess carbohydrates or carbohydrates without a protein and fat, the secretion of insulin is higher and the secretion of glucagon is lower (high insulin-to-glucagon ratio). Consequently, the excess carbohydrates you eat *will be mostly stored as fat.*

When you eat protein with carbohydrates, the secretion of insulin is lower and the secretion of glucagon is higher (low insulin-to-glucagon ratio). The result is that the food you ate will be used to rebuild the body or used as energy; it will not be stored as fat.

Despite this, people believe that eating protein and fat is fattening. But protein and fat actually lower the insulin-to-glucagon ratio, which prevents fat production and storage. Carbohydrates raise the insulin-to-glucagon ratio, which leads to fat production and storage. People also believe that carbohydrates satiate their appetites. But carbohydrates do not satiate you until you have already overeaten.

You Can Overeat Carbohydrates, but You Cannot Overeat Proteins and Good Fats

The body has feedback mechanisms to prevent you from eating too many proteins and fats. But the body does not have this same mechanism to regulate carbohydrates.

True hunger (as opposed to false hunger, which derives from cravings caused by a low serotonin state) is felt when your brain runs out of food and sends a message: "You'd better get me something now because I need sugar for constant energy." If you eat a protein with a fat, first you chew it in your mouth, then it goes to your stomach, where the protein is broken down by enzymes. Protein and fats, along with all the juices that flow in from the stomach, distend the stomach, sending electrical signals to the brain that food has come into the system. Your brain is pacified, having received the signal that food is coming.

Proteins and fats are then released into the small intestine, where a very important hormone called cholecystokinin (CCK) gets secreted from the intestinal wall. CCK goes to the brain and, in turn, announces that food is coming. In addition, CCK also makes your gallbladder contract, secreting bile to help absorb fats. If CCK is over-produced, you will feel nauseated. If you ignore that feeling and you keep eating, you will either become further nauseated or vomit.

To illustrate this process, I ask people to think about how many hard-boiled eggs they can eat at one time. Generally, it is two or three, not six or ten. If you eat too many, you will end up sick to your stomach. Now consider how many bowls of cereal you can eat before you would become sick. Probably many.

People say they enjoy eating carbohydrates because they have that "light" feeling. That "light" feeling is caused by the fact that carbohydrates do not stay in the stomach. They go right through your stomach and into the small intestine. You do not experience stomach distention or the release of CCK in the small intestine, signaling to the brain that you have eaten and that food is coming. Carbohydrates must enter the bloodstream before triggering the release of insulin, which causes a temporary release of serotonin in the brain, signaling the beginning of satiety. Next, the sugar leaves the liver and goes to the brain. At that point your brain-sugar level rises, signaling that you are fully satiated. But carbohydrates have to go through the entire digestive and absorption process before the brain understands it is getting food and stops sending hunger signals. By that time you could have eaten an entire box of cereal. Whereas eating protein and fats signals the brain early on to stop demanding food, with carbohydrates there is no early regulation to say, "Don't eat any more."

When I explain to patients that I want them to cut down on carbohydrates and eat more proteins and fats, they often ask me how much to eat. People are used to calculating and measuring, but one of the purposes of this book is to discourage that practice. I instruct patients to eat as much good fat as their body needs. Examples of good fats are eggs, avocados, flaxseed oil, butter, mayonnaise and olive oil. Examples of bad fats are fried foods and hydrogenated fats. (See chapters 25 and 26 for more on healthy and unhealthy fats.)

Many patients have said to me, "But you don't understand, I crave food all the time. I can eat enormous quantities of food." When I ask them what they are eating, it is always enormous quantities of carbohydrates. If they are really afraid to accept the license to eat, I ask them to try a one-week experiment. For breakfast they are to eat as many eggs as they want, along with nitrate-free sausages, vegetables and one piece of whole-grain toast with butter. For lunch, a chicken Caesar salad with a serving of fruit. Dinner could be fish, chicken or red meat, vegetables lathered in butter, salad with a liberal amount of oil-and-vinegar dressing, one half baked potato (with a lot of butter and sour cream). If they feel hungry between meals, they are to eat a protein, a fat and a carbohydrate, such as a small handful of nuts or mozzarella cheese with a small piece of fruit.

It is my experience that by the end of the week, even patients with very poor eating habits have been able to stay on this healing program. People do not change bad eating or lifestyle habits overnight, however, and some patients are extremely serotonin depleted and cannot stay on this program for even one week. Serotonin plays a major role in how well people are able to adhere to a balanced diet. The brain sends powerful signals that can make willpower ineffective, no matter how much you want to change. Healing takes time and patience as well as balanced serotonin levels, which come about via the gradual regeneration of the metabolism through eating a balanced diet.

One of the benefits of healing is achieving your ideal body composition. Many people are interested in weight loss. People used to fanatically count calories in order to lose weight. In recent years, they have switched to counting fat grams. Chapter 13 will explain why counting calories or fat grams will only lead to more body-fat gain.

Thirteen

Fat Does Not Make You Fat

T he low-fat movement has been in high gear for over ten years now. People have kept strict tabs on their fat intake, believing that "fat makes you fat." At the same time, they have not restricted their carbohydrate consumption at all, believing that, since carbohydrates are fat free, they are "free" calories. Ironically, the only calories that you should keep track of are carbohydrate calories. In fact, the low-fat, high-carbohydrate diet can be the most fattening diet you can go on.

A Calorie Is Not a Calorie

In order to understand how you can gain body fat on a low-fat, high-carbohydrate diet, you must understand what a calorie really is.

Energy from food is called calories. One calorie is actually defined as the amount of energy required to raise one gram of water one degree Celsius. To measure the amount of heat loss of different foods, scientists break the food chemical bonds completely, underwater, and then measure the change in the temperature of the water from the heat generated from these chemical reactions.

To measure the amount of energy in, say, a seven-ounce piece of chicken, you have to break down all the chemical bonds of the proteins and fats into their basic elements of hydrogen, oxygen and carbon.

Scientists have measured the calories in proteins, fats and carbohydrates and have determined that both proteins and carbohydrates have four calories per gram and fat has nine calories per gram. This is where all the confusion began. Because the calorie measurements took place in a test tube where no other factors came into play, scientists wrongly concluded that fat is twice as fattening as proteins and carbohydrates. But this is not true.

To your body, a hundred-calorie snack does not necessarily contain a hundred calories' worth of available energy. The hundred calories reflect only the amount of possible energy that *could* be utilized by your body, depending on what kind of food the snack is. If the snack is composed of carbohydrates, your body has to use the hundred calories for immediate energy or store that energy as fat. But if the snack is made up of protein and fats, your body can use these foods first for building materials (cells, enzymes, hormones and so on), leaving fewer calories to be used as energy or stored as fat.

For example, in a laboratory setting, if you took a seven-ounce piece of chicken (protein and fat) and broke it down into its basic elements of hydrogen, oxygen and carbon, you would find that it contained 380 calories. But when you eat the same piece of chicken, your body does not break the chicken down into its basic elements. The protein and fat in the chicken are only partially broken down into amino acids and fatty acids, which are then used to build new proteins (muscle, hair, skin) and fats (myelin sheaths, cell membranes and hormones).

Since the chicken was never broken down to its basic elements but instead was reconfigured into new proteins and fats, all of the bonds were never actually broken. Therefore, all of the potential energy was never released as it is in a laboratory setting. Because proteins and fats are not broken down into energy and are used instead as building materials, little or none of the proteins and fats goes to fat storage.

Carbohydrates, however, are not used as building materials but instead provide energy that is then used to drive chemical reactions. If the energy derived from carbohydrates is not needed at the moment, carbohydrates are stored as energy, either in ready-energy form as glycogen or in a long-term form as body fat.

These days many experts agree that a calorie-restricted diet is an obsolete approach to body-fat loss. Today we hear that the way to health and fitness is to maintain a strict low-fat diet, counting fat grams. But low-fat diets are even more dangerous to your health than calorie-reduced diets because low-fat diets eliminate two of the most essential nutrient groups.

The following is a description of what would occur in a healthy young adult going on a low-fat diet without restricting carbohydrate calories.

The Low-Fat, High-Carbohydrate Diet

1. In cutting fat out of their diet, most people increase carbohydrate intake. They stop eating eggs for breakfast and instead eat cereal, non-fat milk, a banana, and drink coffee. Lunch is a salad with bread, iced tea or a diet soda. Dinner is pasta with marinara sauce, bread and a glass of wine. Without realizing it, they have drastically reduced their protein intake and increased their carbohydrate and stimulant intake.

   After each high-carbohydrate meal, they feel "light" because carbohydrates travel quickly through the system. They may also feel calmed, since carbohydrates and stimulants cause a temporary release of serotonin, the neurotransmitter in the brain that is responsible for mood.

2. Because the meal was all carbohydrates, it was converted mostly to fat and then used by the cells as energy. However, between

meals, to keep the blood-sugar levels going to the brain tightly controlled, the body draws on its liver glycogen stores. To keep the body in motion, muscle glycogen stores are depleted and those first few pounds fall right off. The person has lost "weight," but that "weight" is not fat.

Unwittingly encouraged by losing those first few pounds, they keep eating the baked potatoes, rice cakes and nonfat pretzels.

3. Because this is a high-carbohydrate diet, they can stay on this diet longer than on a low-calorie diet, since serotonin levels are not depleted as quickly. They continue the low-fat regimen and lose a lot more "weight" than on a low-calorie diet. This is where drastic destruction to metabolism occurs—even more than with a low-calorie diet. To restrict calories, most people generally eat small portions of all the nutrient groups. However, on a low-fat diet, people drastically reduce two of the essential nutrient groups (proteins and fats). The body is then forced to take more proteins and fats from lean body mass.

4. Exercise will cause further "weight loss" as more glycogen and lean body mass are used up, both of which weigh more than fat.

5. Over time they might see body-fat gain around the middle. As you have learned, the midsection is your "insulin meter," indicating prolonged high insulin levels. In this case, the prolonged high insulin has been caused by a high-carbohydrate diet.

6. In an attempt to slow down the self-destruction, metabolic processes begin to slow down.

If they continued on a low-fat, high-carbohydrate diet, they could end up either too thin with a high body-fat composition, or too fat with a high body-fat composition. Regardless of the end "weight," they would not have an ideal body composition.

Why Some People Gain or Lose "Weight" on a Low-Fat, High-Carbohydrate Diet

There are many outcomes when a person goes on a low-fat, high-carbohydrate diet, depending on:

- **Age**
- **Sex hormone levels**
- **Volume of carbohydrates the person eats**
- **Protein and fat intake**
- **Exercise**
- **Level of metabolism when starting the diet**

The following are four examples with six scenarios that could occur on a low-fat, high-carbohydrate diet, depending on the factors listed above.

Person 1 Is a Prepubertal Child with No Sex Hormones

Begins a low-fat, high-carbohydrate diet. Because of this diet, she/he does not go through stages of puberty correctly. Hormone levels stay low and the child remains too thin, without increasing bone and muscle mass that is normally seen in puberty.

Person 2 Is a Healthy Adult with Normal Hormone Levels

This person has never dieted in his/her lifetime but now begins a low-fat, high-carbohydrate diet. He/she will initially lose "weight" and will lose even more "weight" if exercising, thus becoming too thin.

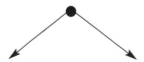

This same person continues a low-fat, high-carbohydrate diet. If sex hormones drop slightly, he/she will gain body fat around the middle.

This same person continues a low-fat, high-carbohydrate diet. If sex hormones drop significantly, he/she will continue to waste away.

Person 3 Has Dieted Chronically All Her/His Life

This person starts off with a lowered metabolism, in addition to imbalanced sex hormone levels. She/he begins a low-fat, high-carbohydrate diet, loses lean body mass and gains body fat.

Person 4 Is Elderly

She/he has no sex hormones. She/he begins a low-fat diet and wastes away.

To achieve optimum health and body composition you must (1) eat a diet that includes proteins, fats and nonstarchy vegetables, and you must eat carbohydrates in accordance with your current metabolism and activity level; (2) manage stress; (3) decrease stimulant use; (4) exercise; and (5) take hormone replacement therapy, if needed.

A common belief is that athletes are the one group that can overeat carbohydrates. But even an athlete like Gordon, whom you will read about in the following chapter, cannot eat a low-fat, high-carbohydrate diet without destroying lean body mass and gaining fat around the midsection.

Fourteen

Gaining Body Fat on a Low-Fat Diet

F at-free or low-fat foods are considered by many to be "free." But in order to eat low-fat foods and avoid gaining a lot of body fat, you would have to be like Gordon, a professional athlete who worked out six to eight hours a day. However, even with all that exercise, Gordon was not in the excellent physical shape he could have been in if he had eaten a balanced diet.

I met Gordon on the tennis court. He was surprised at my strength because he knew that I was too busy to exercise every day. I was surprised about him, too, but in the opposite way. I was astounded by the fat around his middle. He also carried fat around his thighs and buttocks. I knew that he was on the court six hours a day and was a runner, too. It was not a secret that he was obsessed with keeping in shape. Knowing the physiology of the body, and having seen what Gordon was eating at the café in the club, I should not have been as surprised as I was by the shape he was in. But why did he continue to eat a low-fat diet when the results were so plain to see?

When Gordon commented on my strength and muscularity, I said, "I'd be happy to teach you what I know about metabolism and muscle building."

Getting Fat on Eight
Hours of Exercise a Day

Gordon: I wouldn't call myself a professional athlete now, but I played pro tournaments at one time. I was All-American in tennis in college and went on some circuit events. I was very committed. I didn't do anything halfway. I was always the first guy at practice and the last guy to leave. I tried to get whatever edge I could. I graduated in 1970 with a degree in physical education and went on to graduate school, where I studied nutrition.

I started coaching tennis in 1972—primarily competitive athletes— young kids up to touring pros. Not only did I play, I also traveled with some touring pros and top junior players. I played tennis tournaments until I was thirty-eight and still play some benefit events to this day.

To be fit and to be a tennis player you want to be as light as you can so that gravity will have less of an effect on your joints. I was a little over- weight as a kid. I think I carried that image with me. So it was easy to get obsessed about keeping my weight down. I read magazine articles or saw talk shows or listened to aerobic instructors or other quasi-educated people talking about low-fat diets. I don't like to think of myself as being vulnerable to media images that thin is better, but I suppose I am like everyone else.

I cut down to almost no fat in my diet from the early 1980s on. I would take all the skin off of a piece of chicken, look for a little piece of fat and get that off too. I ate a lot of carbs—boxes of crackers, oranges, bananas. For breakfast I ate shredded wheat, blueberries, skim milk and a banana— zero fat. I skipped lunch because I thought, oh, I can't be loaded down at work. At dinner I gorged on carbs. I was hungry and thought, hey, these are free—they're just carbs and don't have any fat. Only fat makes you fat.

In 1988 I was diagnosed with a thyroid disorder—Graves' disease. I was hyperthyroid. For the first six months I was in denial. I went from a resting pulse of 40 to 120. I would sweat even if the weather was cold. I had the shakes. I ate three big meals a day, all carbs, and then went home and had a box of graham crackers with a quart of skim milk because I was so hungry. I couldn't get enough food. I went down to 138 pounds, even though I was eating like a horse.

I went for six years on and off drugs that were supposed to slow down my thyroid. I was supposed to get weaned off the drugs eventually, but instead my dosage was increased. I put on twenty pounds. I didn't fit into my clothes. I was treated with a very conservative dose of radioactive iodine. Six months later, I was hyperthyroid again.

I had gone from bench-pressing 250 pounds to 130. I now know that I had depleted muscle mass—I was definitely weaker. I even stopped playing tennis for a while because I had lost a desire to play because it hurt too much. I would always have shoulder discomfort when I served. I'm forty-eight and thought maybe because I'm over forty, age has finally gotten me. People always told me I looked young. I mean, I got carded when I was forty. So I thought, I look young but, inside, age is catching up to me.

Dr. Schwarzbein: I listened to Gordon's history and explained how we would treat his thyroid problem. Then I directed him to look back at his weight loss when he was first diagnosed with his hyperthyroid condition. He had lost fourteen pounds in a few weeks because an excess of thyroid hormone burns up lean body mass (muscle and bones), which weighs more than fat. Though people are often thrilled to lose weight rapidly, sudden weight loss is never healthy. Losing lean body mass is one way to become insulin resistant. Less muscle mass means fewer insulin receptor doors on cells for insulin to unload sugar. When insulin cannot unload sugar into muscle cells, excess sugar is converted to fat and stored in the available fat cells.

It is physiologically impossible to burn off more than one to two pounds in a week without doing extreme damage to your metabolism. For Gordon to have lost that much weight meant he had lost not just fat but muscle. This holds true for anyone on a fasting weight-loss program— liquid fasts or low-calorie diets. If you lose weight quickly, you have lost not only fat but also muscle mass.

Muscle mass is the backbone of your metabolic rate. Muscle mass uses more energy than the rest of the tissues. The more muscle mass you have, the higher your metabolism, and the less muscle mass, the lower the metabolism. If only bathroom scales could tell how much muscle mass we lose versus how much fat we lose! But of course scales measure total weight, not body composition, which is very misleading and often encourages more dieting—setting you up for more body-fat gain.

I explained to Gordon that rapid weight loss indicates something is wrong in the body. Rapid weight loss can occur during periods of malnutrition, extreme dieting, illness, stress or extended physical activity. In addition to medical treatment, proper nutrition is key to preventing more muscle burning and in turning the metabolism around. Gordon was a worst-case scenario—a person with a hyperthyroid condition who ate a low-fat, low-protein, high-carbohydrate diet and who skipped meals and worked out excessively. This was an equation for disaster. He had lost a lot of muscle mass rapidly and had become weak while also suffering from body aches and pains. He was destroying himself rapidly.

What Happens When You Eat a Low-Fat, High-Carbohydrate Diet

1. When you eat a low-fat diet, you reduce your intake of protein and fat and increase your consumption of carbohydrates.
2. The digestion of carbohydrates results in high levels of blood sugar being delivered to your liver.
3. Excess blood sugar is converted to triglycerides (fat) and is used either as energy by the body or stored as fat.
4. Continuing to eat an excess of carbohydrates sends a steady supply of blood sugar to the brain, keeping it satisfied.
5. The absence of adequate proteins and fats in the diet forces the body to recruit these vital nutrients by breaking down its own muscle and bone mass.
6. Years of eating a low-fat diet will result in the interior rearrangement of your body's composition. Muscle mass will shrink, bones will become less dense and body fat will increase.

We can use Gordon's case as an accelerated example of what is going on with many people today because excess thyroid hormone quickly wastes lean body mass as does eating a low-fat, high-carbohydrate diet. Anyone eating a low-fat, low-protein, high-carbohydrate diet will end up losing lean body mass and replacing it with fat. Symptoms such as Gordon experienced—decreased energy levels, muscle aches and pains, and body-fat gain around the middle—are typical results of a low-fat, high-carbohydrate diet.

I explained to Gordon that high levels of insulin from a diet high in carbohydrates keep fat in the fat cells. But if he ate more protein and fat and reduced his carbohydrate and stimulant consumption, he would steadily lose body fat whether he continued to work out or not. Rebuilding his lean body mass would increase cells with insulin receptor doors to accept sugar, which would increase his metabolism and thus heal his insulin resistance. I cautioned Gordon not to overeat carbohydrates even if he was exercising more than usual. There is never a good time to overeat carbohydrates.

Even very athletic people should strive to keep their meals balanced. People believe that they can eat a bowl of pasta to "carbo-load" before exercising and that they will "burn" it off. It is true that you can burn off excess sugar as energy. However, you cannot burn off the excess insulin that has been secreted to match the high sugar. Once insulin levels increase to a higher than normal level, damage begins to occur in your metabolism. High insulin levels destroy the metabolism by setting off a multitude of chain reactions that disrupt all other hormones and biochemical cellular reactions. This leads to increased inflammatory responses, cellular growth, blood clotting and insulin resistance.

Furthermore, people confuse energy with stamina. To become a high-performing athlete you must build lean body mass by eating sufficient proteins and fats. A well-conditioned body will perform at its optimum. You cannot simply load up on sugar and expect high performance. There are many studies that prove that athletes who eat a balanced diet outperform those who eat a high-carbohydrate diet.

The most widely held misconception is that carbohydrates "energize" you. But energy from carbohydrates can be used only if needed, otherwise you will convert the excess energy into fat, which will be stored. The most obvious signs of carbohydrate overconsumption are afternoon fatigue and body-fat gain on normal amounts of food.

Gordon: Dr. Schwarzbein took over my thyroid treatment. I was concerned about my physical shape too. She explained to me what metabolism was. She said, "Let's make your metabolism work."

I said, "I'm going to try the program and see what happens." From the day that Dr. Schwarzbein explained the program to me, I didn't eat any more sugar. That's the way I am. I can't see doing it halfway. If I do it all the way, then I'll see the real results. I started eating protein and made myself eat three times a day. At first I resisted fat because I was so brainwashed. I cut the carbs way down. I cut out sodas and juices and fruits. But I still couldn't see eating butter. Eventually she got through to me, explaining that the body needs fat for hormone production.

It's been fourteen months now. I have more energy and I'm seeing most of my strength come back. I'm playing tennis again. Now when I run my legs don't hurt afterwards. I weigh 160, but the weight is different. I eat right and I don't care about how much I weigh. I care how I feel and how my clothes fit.

I feel much better and I see the potential to do even better yet. Because of the combined damage of my thyroid condition and what I was eating, I had no building blocks to build biceps, deltoids, abdominal muscles or to keep connective tissue strong. Now that I understand the physiology, I realize that bodybuilders have known it all along. Go to Gold's Gym and ask the strongest guys what they are eating, and they may say five thousand calories a day—and much of it is protein.

Dr. Schwarzbein: Because Gordon had eaten a low-fat diet for over ten years, he will not reach his goal of optimum health and his ideal body composition overnight. Healing takes time.

Like Gordon, you can change your metabolism, but you need to give your body the necessary nourishment to do so. Everyone, not only athletes, should be trying to build lean body stores on a daily basis. We are all

Why Carbo-Loading Is Damaging

You eat excess carbohydrates

↓

Mouth

↓

Small intestine

↓

High sugar reaches portal vein

↓

Pancreas secretes large amounts of insulin

↓

Liver

Some sugar is used for immediate energy. But the high insulin levels have already caused metabolic damage.

Some sugar is stored in the form of glycogen. But the high insulin levels have already caused metabolic damage.

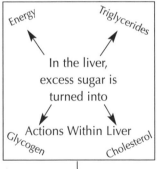

In the liver, excess sugar is turned into

Actions Within Liver

Excess sugar is turned into fat for storage and/or energy. But the high insulin levels have already caused metabolic damage.

Excess sugar is turned into cholesterol. But the high insulin levels have already caused metabolic damage.

↓

Tightly regulated amounts of sugar are sent to the brain and body. But the high insulin levels have already caused metabolic damage.

born with the potential to form strong healthy tissues, but the body needs help to accomplish this. It needs proteins and fats from your diet to use as the building material for structures such as cells, cell membranes, hormones, neurotransmitters, enzymes, tissues and organs.

Robert, whom you read about in chapter 2, wasted away on a low-fat, high-carbohydrate, low-protein, low-calorie diet. Gordon lost lean body tissue and gained body fat on a low-fat, low-protein, high-carbohydrate diet. Both Robert and Gordon deprived their bodies of necessary proteins and fats. Their bodies were forced to look for protein and fat within the body to keep metabolic processes going. When your body tears itself down, premature aging begins. At the same time, Gordon's low-fat, high-carbohydrate, low-protein diet promoted body-fat storage around the midsection, which is why I call the midsection the "insulin meter."

You learned in chapter 7 that people can initially see improvements in their cholesterol profiles by going on a low-fat diet and exercise regimen. But, by losing lean body mass, eventually they will see those results reversed. In addition to cholesterol profiles, people can see initial body-fat loss and improvements in high blood pressure as well. Because some people have experienced initial "success" on a low-fat diet, the misconceptions about fat have become ingrained in our society. It is sometimes difficult to dispel those beliefs—especially when a doctor advises a patient to eat low-fat, as I did early on in my practice with Charles, whom you will read about in chapter 15.

Fifteen

Dispelling Low-Fat Beliefs

C harles was one of my first patients when I began my medical practice. I had just finished nine years of medical training in which I was taught that eliminating dietary fat was the way to stay fit and healthy, so I had asked him to keep his fat intake low and he followed my instructions well.

Soon afterward, the "cheaters" on this program made me rethink everything I had learned in medical school. (As you read in the Introduction, the cheaters were the patients who dramatically increased their fat consumption over what I had prescribed.) Through the results of the cheaters, I discovered that my low-fat prescription was wrong. Unfortunately, Charles was not one of the cheaters, and it was nearly impossible to get him to begin eating fat again.

Charles: In 1987, at age fifty-nine, I remember my doctor telling me that my blood sugar was pretty high the morning I went in for my annual checkup, but he thought that I was all right. Eventually, though, we found out I had diabetes.

I was sent to a young internist to treat my diabetes. He prescribed the ADA diet. Pastas were fine, bananas were fine, potatoes were fine.

This went on for four years. I was getting no results at all. In fact, I was gradually dying on the vine, to tell you the honest truth. My health was deteriorating badly. I ran a plumbing business. I would have to come home in the afternoon and literally lay down and take a rest so I could go out and finish my work. My triglycerides, as I remember, were 1045. Normal is around 100. My blood sugar was completely off the chart. I was told I had a premature cataract because of this high blood sugar. I'm five feet, nine inches, and I weighed 210: overweight—or six inches too short. My health was deteriorating. I couldn't see it in myself, but my wife Emily saw it.

Emily and I first saw Diana Schwarzbein in 1991. At our first meeting, Dr. Schwarzbein looked at this diet I was on and nearly fell out of her chair. She said, "This is outrageous. I can't believe this is still going on."

During the visit, she said, "If you'll go with my program for six months, we can make a different person out of you." I could see the diet coming down. I could see everything that I wanted to eat going right out the door. She said, "If you don't want to go with my program for six months you might as well pay the cashier and leave." I laugh about that to this day.

Well, my wife is a five-star general. I thought that between the two of them they had conspired to kill me. It was a tremendously bold move on both of their parts.

Emily: After the first appointment with Dr. Schwarzbein, I went through the freezer, the refrigerator and the cupboards and threw out everything I could get my hands on. Pancake mix. Canned goods. Packaged macaroni and cheese. All processed foods. I threw out boxes and boxes of food. We had practically nothing left in the cupboards. We became vegetable eaters.

Charles: We were strictly on a vegetable routine. And at the time my cholesterol was so high that Dr. Schwarzbein jerked me off of most fatty stuff. Absolutely no sugar and also very low in other carbohydrates.

She said, "You don't need your blood sugar medication. Your diet will take care of your high blood sugar." From the very first day, we saw a result in the blood sugar. Also, within a three-week period I went from three blood pressure pills a day down to none at all. My cholesterol also started to drop, and my triglycerides went from 1045 to the 165 range.

How You Can Get Good *Initial* Results by Eliminating Dietary Fats

Unfortunately, I met Charles before my nutritional program was fully developed. Because I had advised him to reduce his fat and carbohydrate intake, Charles, like many Americans thought, *if less is good, then none is better.*

The rapid drop in his blood sugars enabled him to stop his diabetes medicine. His blood pressure came down, so we tapered him off of his blood-pressure medicines. Next, his body used his fat stores for energy, which caused him to lose body fat and improved his cholesterol levels.

All this sounds great, and these kinds of testimonials are exactly why many people believe the claims that eating a low-fat diet will make them trim and healthy. But let me explain why the low-fat diet works initially, then backfires. If you reduce fats, the most concentrated energy source, from your diet, your body will use all incoming sugar and fat as energy—which lowers overall blood-sugar and insulin levels.

Insulin is a hormone responsible for fat production, blood-volume changes and cholesterol production. If you lower insulin levels you will lose fat, have lower blood pressure and lower cholesterol levels. That still sounds good.

But as you learned in chapter 1, when you deprive your body of fat you also deprive your body of protein; this decreases your lean body mass. Decreased muscle mass means that there are fewer cells with insulin receptor doors to accept sugar. At this state, your metabolism has slowed down which means that your energy requirement is much lower than it used to be, and any excess sugar must be converted into fat and stored in available fat cells—this is early insulin resistance.

While some people experience great initial results from a low-fat diet, they eventually experience a decline in health. They gain body fat, see abnormal cholesterol numbers, increased blood pressure, and they may develop any of the degenerative diseases of aging.

Since the destruction from eating a low-fat diet occurs over many years, the correlation is not an easy one to make. People tend to blame their decline on genetics instead of on their eating habits. "My dad was overweight too." Or, "High blood pressure runs in my family." Unfortunately, most people accept this fatalistic argument. People are told that poor health is genetic, so they simply tolerate illness and decreased quality of life as their lot.

Dr. Schwarzbein: As Charles returned for follow-up visits, I recognized that he was wasting away on his starvation diet of only proteins and vegetables and that his cholesterol levels were starting to climb again. By the time I had seen him a few times, I had come to the conclusion that the human physiology requires fats to maintain normal cholesterol levels. I explained that I had been very wrong in telling him to cut dietary fat, that dietary fat was essential for healing and to maintaining good health.

However, my talks did little to sway his opinion of the benefit of the low-fat diet. For twenty years Charles had heard that he should eliminate fats from his diet, and he had experienced initial great results in doing so. To make matters worse, *I* had initially told him that very same thing!

During each subsequent office visit, I explained that I had been wrong in instructing him to reduce his fat intake. I explained to both Charles and Emily that fats are good and that dietary fat was crucial to his staying healthy. I encouraged him to eat *as much butter, eggs and oils as he wanted.* After every visit, I believed that finally I had gotten through to him. But the next time I saw him, I would realize that I had not been as successful as I thought.

I explained to Charles that in addition to losing body fat, he had lost a dangerous amount of lean body mass as well because he was not eating essential dietary fats. He needed to think of dietary fat as the food group that would heal him after my mistaken advice. It was vitally important to his health that he begin eating unlimited amounts of fat to regain his lean body mass. Without dietary fat he would waste away even further.

Charles and Emily are classic examples of how fixed our society's mind-set has become regarding the claims of the low-fat movement.

Charles: For a long time, I was kicked clear off fat because Dr. Schwarzbein was trying to bring my weight down. My weight went from 210 to 150 pounds. It was such a quick slide that she put me on some other fats and stuff like that because my food window was so small you couldn't crawl through it. When she got my weight down she started letting me eat fat. I'm totally unrestricted as far as fat goes now. When Dr. Schwarzbein put fats back into my diet, it was like manna from heaven.

I eat real butter, real sour cream, real whipping cream, real cream cheese. I eat hamburger meat and steaks. Now, I'm not a big steak eater anymore at all, but at one time in my life, if I went out to dinner and didn't have a steak I felt totally gypped. Now I get along quite comfortably with a nice piece of fish or chicken. But when she increased my fats—my goodness, I could eat a sausage once in a while with my eggs. It was wonderful.

Dr. Schwarzbein: I was glad when Charles finally put dietary fat back in his diet. I am sorry that he never understood the real reasons I asked him to eat dietary fat. He and Emily held on to the popular belief that low fat causes good "weight loss." Because Charles lost so much weight initially on a low-fat, low-carbohydrate diet, it only served to confirm their beliefs. He never understood that his weight loss was caused by losing lean body mass, not body fat.

Charles: I can't believe how good I feel at sixty-eight years old this month. I can work any young man into the ground. Dr. Schwarzbein put me on an exercise routine. At first I could not understand it. I told her, "I work hard all day." And she said, "But that's not good enough." You've got to have this *thump, thump, thump, thump*. So I got on an exercise routine. Bought one of these stationary bikes that I hate. I wasn't a walker at that time. Now I'll get out rain or shine and do my walking every night. I walk two miles, and I'm not breathing hard.

Dr. Schwarzbein: Exercise was extremely important in Charles's case since he had come to me being diabetic, which is the last stage of insulin resistance. Exercise helps the body burn off excessive stored energy in cells. It also increases lean body mass; both of these things increase insulin receptor doors.

Charles and Emily told me that they both eat the same way now. Everyone in the family is affected when one person changes his or her eating habits. When one family member incorporates dietary fats and proteins and cuts down on carbohydrates, this change is very good for the whole family. If only everyone could be as willing as Charles and Emily were! I would be very happy if everyone who came to see me did what Emily did that first day when she went through cupboards and threw out all the high-sugar and processed foods.

While I often encourage people to "do the best they can," diabetics—who have the worst metabolism—have to try their best to achieve perfection when it comes to nutrition and lifestyle habits. Even though I stress perfection in my program, you can see how it does not translate to the real-life situations depicted in this book. However, as you can also see, while people are not perfect, they can enjoy results by simply making a few changes. Anything you do to improve your eating and lifestyle habits, especially getting off your low-fat diet, will improve your heath.

Good health progresses on a cellular level. Everyone can take charge of his or her health and begin to heal poor metabolism. Balanced nutrition heals you physically, but it also calms the "noise" in your head that demands carbohydrates and stimulants. Chronic dieting, carbohydrate craving, bingeing and addictions can be corrected when the body is properly nourished. Part V shares the stories of several women, including myself, who overcame various forms of eating disorders.

PART V

Eating Disorders

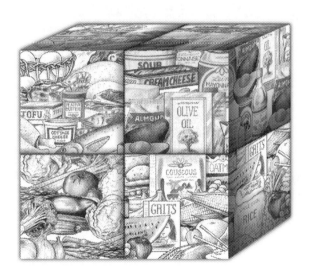

Sixteen

Diet Scams

Y ou may not be convinced that you should go off your low-fat
diet. You have heard for twenty years that eliminating fat is the
way to good health. And now you are reading that a low-fat diet
is bad for you. What are you going to believe when the "experts" are
always changing their minds? One day it is, "Eat this," the next year it
is, "No, don't eat this, eat that."

When diet and nutrition fads come and go, for most of us it is
nothing more than a minor annoyance, at worst an inconvenience.
But for some, false claims, diet scams, and misconceptions about
health and nutrition can be devastating. Not only emotionally, but
physically as well.

One of my patients, Elizabeth, came to my office with her husband
to discuss her infertility problem. Elizabeth was a poised young
woman in her early thirties. The following story chronicles her
twenty-five years of heartache as she struggled with her weight by
counting calories and following liquid and low-fat diets.

Victim of the Diet Industry

Elizabeth: I swam competitively from age five and also played tennis and soccer. By the time I was twelve, I was a big girl. But in 1973, people weren't used to girls being big, muscular or athletic. My own family didn't seem to notice that there were a lot of other big people in the family; instead they focused way too much on my size.

Growing up, I would have never been characterized as the chubby outsider. I was a star athlete. I had steady boyfriends from the time I was twelve years old. From the outside I was a totally normal, athletic girl— always part of the "in crowd." The obsession was inside my head.

Once, in junior high, I needed a pair of jeans for a camping trip. I couldn't fit into anything. Clothes were cut for skinny kids. If I didn't wear jeans, the option was Danskin stretch pants. I ended up not going on the trip.

Mom said, "Don't worry, we'll do Weight Watchers!"

In junior high school, Mom would pick me up to come home for lunch and I just hated it. It was all about deprivation, you know. My brother and sister didn't have weight problems. We'd go out to have dinner and when it came to dessert it was, "Okay, everyone but Elizabeth." Food became covert. Here Mom was making all these Weight Watchers meals and picking me up for lunch and really trying to do it right, and I'm riding my bike to the store for candy and hiding it.

All my friends were getting their periods. I didn't start until I was eighteen. Then I would only have one every four to eight months. But nobody seemed worried, so I didn't worry either. I had enough to think about.

From twelve to eighteen, I did Weight Watchers a bunch of times and then went to The Weight Place. One diet included weekly shots. Later on, I found out they had something to do with cow urine. I lost some weight on that diet. Of course, I gained it back. Deprivation would set in, and I would sneak off to eat. Food became a hidden, shameful thing to me.

Weight Watchers, the shots, everything I tried was about low-calorie intake. Calories equaled fat. Weight Watchers let you have sugar things and carbo things. That wasn't the issue. The amount of calories you took in was the obsession at that time. Weighing portions on a stupid scale.

From the time I started doing all those diet things, I was either hating myself because I was fat or hating myself because I wasn't dieting. There was no peaceful period. Ever. Unless I was starving and depriving myself in some way, I didn't feel like a worthy human. I assumed that every other girl in the world was starving herself, too. If you went out on a date and ate salad, then what a desirable catch you were!

As a senior in high school I lost thirty pounds at The Weight Place. Then I put on fifty pounds during my freshman year in college. Being tall, I can gain a lot of weight and not look that much different. But by my senior year in college I was another fifty pounds overweight. I went on the Diet Center diet and lost it all. I was the thinnest I have ever been. I was beautiful. Being thin meant I was the sexual being that men wanted. Still, I was miserable. It was the same cycle replaying itself. Hating myself because I couldn't relax. Obsessing about everything I put in my mouth. My life felt fractured and out of control. My weight, my obsession with sneaking food and eating food, the panic attacks, what I looked like and not having periods. All that ruled my life.

Near the end of my senior year, my two closest friends were killed in a car accident. I couldn't focus on being the sexual, fun girl anymore. I was in so much grief and pain. Food was my coping mechanism. Food was calming. Heavy carbo foods. Ice cream. Breads. They were like drugs— soothing. I put on a lot of weight. Body size became a hiding place.

I got married when I was twenty-four. I lost weight for the wedding. My husband and I bought a Diet Center franchise together. I got very thin again and, to my great surprise, I got pregnant. My periods had always been so sporadic that getting pregnant was a shock. I loved being pregnant because I did not have anyone monitoring my food. I was free.

I had my daughter when I was twenty-five. Afterward, I did a liquid-fast diet, the ultimate body blower. I lost seventy pounds and I was absolutely stunning. But any semblance of metabolism that I had left was wrecked. At the time, all I cared about was that I went from okay to gorgeous.

We sold the Diet Center, and then I became a disc jockey with a morning radio show. My marriage started to fall apart. Something had to give. I didn't want to give up my marriage. What gave was the food. I retreated to the safe place. My weight crept from 150 pounds to 260 pounds, the heaviest I'd ever been. When I started putting on weight, the people I worked with were appalled. I was so popular before because I looked so good for public appearances. All of a sudden I didn't represent the radio station anymore. Of course, I ended up leaving the station.

But at this over-the-top weight I couldn't get a job to save my soul. I finally got hired by Campfire Boys and Girls. The woman who hired me said, "I've noticed that larger women are the best employees, so I hire big women." I was shocked. I didn't see myself that way.

Dr. Schwarzbein: As I listened to Elizabeth's history, I knew exactly why this athletic woman had gained so much body fat. I believed that she was not "pigging out" in the back closet. People assume that because a person is overweight, they are also overnourished. Nothing could be further from the truth. When an overweight person comes to see me, the first diagnosis I make is malnourishment. The word *malnutrition* conjures up pictures of people in concentration camps or victims of famine. Robert, who wasted away on a low-fat, low-protein, low-calorie diet, suffered from malnutrition, and so did Elizabeth, even though she had gained an excessive amount of body fat.

Millions of Years of Genetics Can Work Against You

Remember, we have the same physiology as prehistoric humans. Because food was not always as available as it is today, the prehistoric human physiology adapted to the feast-and-famine environment by evolving an insulin-directed fat-storage system. It is an insulin-directed system because insulin directs nutrients and fat into the cells. This system enabled humans to store food as fat as insurance against future times of need.

When prehistoric humans went without food for long periods of time their bodies readjusted, so the next time they gorged during a plentiful season, their insulin levels went to a higher level than before.

That translated to more fat storage. More body fat was a good thing because it meant that they could survive in lean times. When they made it through a long winter by using the fat stored in their bodies, it meant another year when they could produce offspring and perpetuate their DNA.

Modern humans have never lost this fat-storage system even though we no longer need it now that food is readily available year-round. And although this physiology worked well for prehistoric humans, it backfires today because we have gotten so far away from the food chain and, more important, because food is more available and excesses have become the norm.

Because of the insulin-directed, fat-storage system, if a person has been undereating, yo-yo dieting or eating the wrong foods most of his or her life, that person will be more prone to store energy in the form of increased body fat. Most people go on diets to get trim and healthy, but instead end up suffering from malnutrition, which, in turn, makes them fat and unhealthy or thin and unhealthy.

Low-calorie diets supply well below the normal nutrient-intake levels required to meet the body's needs for ongoing metabolic processes. Low-calorie diets always fail to keep body fat off. Most of you know this because you have tried to restrict calories to lose fat and have failed. You think it is because you do not have self-control. But there are other more important physiological factors that prevent you from losing body fat and keeping it off, especially when you try to accomplish body-fat loss on a low-calorie diet.

In earlier chapters you read about the process of low-calorie/low-fat dieting and then low-fat dieting alone. Low-calorie dieting may not be as popular as it once was. However, many people still suffer the ill effects of having dieted this way. I will take you through the process of a calorie-restricted diet to show you how your prehistoric physiology reacts by storing more fat every time you go through a "lean" time (diet). Below is a description of what would occur in a healthy young adult going on a low-calorie diet. Note that, as you age, the metabolism changes, and this scenario would also change.

Why You Cannot Lose Body Fat on a Calorie-Restricted Diet

1. Two hours after eating, your body has used or stored the available sugar energy from your last meal. Because your body needs constant refueling, it begins to need more energy at this time.

2. It takes energy from liver glycogen to keep your blood-sugar level tightly controlled. At the same time, the muscles use their glycogen for energy.

3. As your glycogen stores are being used, some fat is burned off as well. Suddenly you see weight loss! You can lose up to nine pounds in the first week of dieting because glycogen weighs much more than fat.

   But this is the stage of low-calorie dieting when most people lose the battle. With the glycogen stores depleted, it is difficult for the liver to regulate blood-sugar supply to the brain. Within one to two weeks, your body demands the sugar it has been deprived of. At this point, you resume eating more calories. Or, if you have amazing willpower, usually aided by some form of stimulant, you continue your low-calorie diet.

4. If you continue with the low-calorie diet, your body is forced to take material from bones and muscles to keep your brain and kidneys going.

   But you do not recognize that you are burning lean body mass. All you care about at this point is that you are starting to weigh less on the scale. You keep looking at the scale, thinking this is the way to go. You continue a low-calorie diet.

5. Your body continues to burn fat, too. But the fat loss is minimal compared to the destruction that is occurring in your muscle and bone mass.

> *It is impossible to lose more than two pounds of body fat a week*—even if you have a high-performing metabolism and exercise rigorously. This is a very important fact and one that is frequently lied about by the diet industry. If you are on a diet and losing weight faster than two pounds a week (after the first week), you are losing lean body mass, not fat.

6. Your metabolism begins to slow down, preventing your body from using too much muscle and bone mass as building materials.

7. You are now down to your goal weight and/or cannot continue dieting any longer. At this point, you have less lean body mass and a lower metabolism. When you resume eating *normal amounts* of food, you gain back all the lean body mass you lost, plus more body fat. Because you are young, your metabolism goes back to where it was before you began your diet. Now, however, you have more body fat than you started out with.

8. Because you gained back more body fat than you had before you started your diet, you are inclined to diet again. This time you resolve to do it better. You blame your increased body fat on your lack of willpower—you did not restrict enough calories during your diet, or did not stay on your diet long enough, or when you resumed eating "normally" you ate too much.

9. So you diet again and the same thing happens. You have now gotten on the "yo-yo" diet track.

The up-and-down effects of yo-yo dieting occur because every time you diet you lose more lean body mass and deprive your body of the nutrients needed to maintain a healthy hormone system. By the time you have gone on multiple diets, losing and regaining "weight," a major shift has occurred in your body composition as well as in your hormone systems. This is compounded because you have gotten older. Every time you diet, you have less potential for rebuilding muscle, less potential for burning body fat and more potential for storing body fat.

Dieting upsets the balance the human body needs for constant nourishment. When you diet, your body perceives a famine and starts to slow down metabolic functions in an attempt to conserve its own lean body mass. If you diet drastically, with liquid fasts or five-hundred-calorie weight-reduction programs, the damage occurs faster.

Elizabeth's radical weight gain was the result of all her years of undereating (famine/dieting). Ask anyone who is one hundred to two hundred pounds overweight, and you will hear a similar scenario. There are very few exceptions to this rule about weight gain—mainly cases of inborn errors of metabolism, and the children in these cases have excessive body fat well before puberty. Everyone else begins life with the same potential metabolism.

Elizabeth: I got into the goddess movement, becoming friends with women who were all body sizes, who were absolutely beautiful. I saw a whole different way of being.

For the next two years I ate whatever I wanted, guilt free. I had to heal thirty-year-old wounds of equating my worth as a person with what I ate. Then I decided to become a vegetarian. It seemed like the healthy, natural thing to do.

My husband and I had been trying to get pregnant since my daughter was about two, and I was concerned about not having periods. So I went to fertility specialists and endocrinologists. They all focused on my weight and told me to go on a low-fat, high-carbo diet. I'd say, "That's what I'm eating. I'm a vegetarian."

They'd say, "Well, you need to exercise."

I've always exercised. So I'd reply, "I swim and walk."

They'd go, "Yeah, uh-huh."

They were disgusted by me. I was the pig of the world and they couldn't stand dealing with me. I'd walk out of doctors' offices thinking, "You have no idea how beautiful I am."

It was the most painful, abusive period of my life. I was taking the best care of myself according to the American Medical Association, and I was being treated like I was eating cakes by the pound. The only reason I didn't go crazy was because my husband was so great. Even during the times our marriage was under strain, my husband never pressured me about my weight.

My parents were going nuts, constantly saying, "You need to do something! You need to diet!"

I told them, "This is what dieting did to me. I'm never dieting again."

I weighed 293 pounds when I went to see Dr. Schwarzbein in December 1994. She looked at me and said, "I can help you." She listened to me and nodded her head and believed what I told her. She validated my experience. "You've been trying to do everything right," she said, "but you've had the wrong information."

Dr. Schwarzbein told me to turn 180 degrees from what I believed to be true: eat fats and protein and less carbs.

Afterwards I said, "This is another crock. This is another food fad and I'm the guinea pig. Two years from now they're going to say, 'Oh, you know, we screwed up. You shouldn't be doing this after all.'"

Dr. Schwarzbein wanted me to write down everything I ate. Everything hit me wrong. I kept thinking, "I'm going to do this and lose weight and gain it back. Or I'm going to eat all this fat and have a heart attack."

Dr. Schwarzbein: I explained to Elizabeth that she had a condition called Stein-Leventhal syndrome (SLS). SLS is a clinical condition of abnormal body-fat gain, infertility (abnormal menstrual cycles), acne and increased facial hair (all four symptoms do not necessarily occur together). SLS occurs only in women, and is associated with insulin resistance and high androgen levels.

Insulin secretion increases the production and secretion of androgens from the adrenal gland, where they are made. Androgens are the "male" hormones that both men and women have. Women as well as men need the right amount of these hormones for normal body physiology. But if androgens are overproduced in a woman they can lead to increased facial hair, acne and irregular periods and infertility as well as body-fat gain around the middle. That is why SLS patients carry their excess fat mainly around the middle, as men do.

Elizabeth's symptoms of SLS were clear. I explained that I had success-fully treated other woman with SLS through nutrition and exercise. In addition, some women also need hormone replacement therapy, but that did not turn out to be the case with Elizabeth.

Prolonged high insulin levels were either the cause of her Stein-Leventhal syndrome or exacerbated it. High insulin levels are caused by stress, dieting, caffeine, alcohol, aspartame, tobacco, steroids, lack of exer-cise, stimulant and other recreational drugs, excessive and/or unnecessary thyroid-replacement therapy and all over-the-counter and prescription drugs. But the number-one cause of increased insulin levels in Elizabeth was a low-fat, high-carbohydrate diet coupled with chronic dieting. In order to reverse the SLS, she had to reduce her carbohydrate consump-tion, especially man-made carbohydrates, and eat more food.

Being a very bright woman, she asked a lot of questions. I understood that she was fed up with diets. I knew the only reason she would consider any new approach was that she wanted to get pregnant again. Still, I was surprised at her resistance. Elizabeth had counted calories and fat grams for so long that asking her to do yet another "diet" seemed irrational to her. I reassured her that this was not a fad diet. This was a clinical program to help patients alter their abnormal metabolism. The healing program was designed to renourish her while lowering insulin levels, which would lower androgen levels, and cure her SLS, enabling her to get pregnant.

Stress and Infertility

Human beings are supposed to eat from the four basic nutrient groups because, as part of the food chain, we are made out of these nutrients. When humans get away from nutritional and lifestyle bal-ance, our systems break down, causing hormonal imbalances. In

Elizabeth's case, chronic dieting made it impossible for her to get pregnant.

Modern humans' low-calorie and low-fat dieting has triggered an increase of infertility. In fact, infertility is one of the diseases of civilization that corresponds to the rise in popularity of the low-fat movement during the last twenty years. This rise of infertility is directly related to the insulin-directed fat-storage system that evolved in prehistoric humans to perpetuate DNA (the human race).

This may seem confusing, since the insulin-directed fat-storage system caused prehistoric humans to store fat and thus survive. Indeed, fat storage was essential to getting prehistoric humans through times of famine. But remember, unlike modern humans, prehistoric humans procreated only during peak sex-hormone years and during times of plenty. More important, between times of famine prehistoric humans did not work out excessively and eat nonfoods. It is a safe bet that during times of plenty, prehistoric humans took full advantage of many fresh meats, fish, fruits, nuts and berries. Eating their fill of fresh, unadulterated foods gave prehistoric humans the resources to produce balanced sex hormones and thus procreate.

In modern times, restricting food is a man-made stressor because food is now generally accessible. Eating a low-calorie diet signals stress to your body. If your body is stressed by not eating correctly, your sex hormones will become imbalanced, causing your reproductive system to shut down. Stress indicates that it is not a good time to bring offspring into the world because you might not be around to breastfeed and take care of your young. If there is not enough food, or if there is a possibility that you are going to die during the childbearing process, your body interferes with the ability to conceive. This is evident by the fact that women stop ovulating when their bodies are not nourished.

We are trying to have babies later on in life, which is a major factor in the rise in infertility. The most ideal physiological time for childbearing is between the ages of fifteen and twenty-five. Although humans were not intended to bear children later on in life, it is still physiologically possible to do so as long as you maintain a healthy metabolism. The difference between a healthy and unhealthy metabolism is *the age of your metabolism*. Because everything you have done to your body since birth contributes to the age of your metabolism, a woman of twenty-five can have an older metabolism than a woman of thirty-five, depending on how those two women have eaten and how they have lived their lives.

Dr. Schwarzbein: Fortunately, Elizabeth was still chronologically young and, even more important, had not irreparably harmed her metabolism. To begin reversing her insulin resistance I recommended that she begin the healing program by cutting out most carbohydrates. I asked her to eat meats, poultry, fish, good fats, nonstarchy vegetables and a very small amount of carbohydrates. This healing program decreases high insulin levels, subsequently decreasing androgen levels. In addition to curing her Stein-Leventhal syndrome, Elizabeth would steadily lose body fat on a diet low in carbohydrates. This occurs because a decreased consumption of carbohydrates causes the insulin-to-glucagon ratios to decrease, and the body uses fat stored in the fat cells for energy. Even more important, Elizabeth needed to eat more good fats because eating fat lowers insulin secretion.

However, I cautioned her that even if she was eager to lose body fat quickly, reducing carbohydrates to zero would not be healthy. The goal is to achieve optimum health and ideal body composition by keeping insulin levels balanced. Rapidly lowering insulin levels by dropping carbohydrates to zero would likely lead to decreased production of serotonin, causing fatigue, depression, insomnia, increased appetite and headaches. In other words, dropping carbohydrates to zero would only create other problems, perpetuating an unhealthy metabolism. When insulin levels are kept too low (by overexercising and not eating enough food), you will waste away and can suffer from a number of conditions such as depression, fatigue, insomnia and rapid bone loss.

Elizabeth could achieve the positive results (body-fat loss, improvement in mood, lowering of cholesterol, higher energy level and so on) on a diet sufficient in proteins, fats, nonstarchy vegetables with slightly less than enough carbohydrates to match her current metabolism and activity level.

I also recommend reducing stress, caffeine, alcohol, nicotine and aspartame, all of which cause insulin to rise dramatically. Exercise and eating good fats (flaxseed oil, butter, olive oil, for example) and fiber help insulin levels to normalize.

Elizabeth: I started eating according to Dr. Schwarzbein's program, and after the first month my weight and cholesterol dropped. I lost fifty pounds in nine months, going from 293 to 243 pounds. Then I got a period! The first one in four years. Two months later I got a positive pregnancy test.[1]

I've been on the program for a year and six months. I've lost seventy pounds so I am at 223 pounds now. I'm still losing, even though I'm five months pregnant. I'm healthy and the baby is healthy and my blood pressure is low. I look better than I did when I was pregnant with my first daughter. It's totally different. I'm not on a diet anymore. This is not a diet. It's as if my body is a chemistry experiment, and I finally understand how it works. I'm never really hungry anymore. It's an amazing thing to not be hungry and still be okay with myself.

I understand now that my perfect weight then was 180. I was a curvy, busty girl who became a curvy, busty woman. But all my best girlfriends weighed 130 to 135. My mother weighed 130. Focusing on the number on the scale caused so much emotional damage and drove me to such desperate lengths in dieting. The other side of the story resulted from all the dieting, especially the liquid diet. After that, I couldn't weigh 180 pounds anymore. Nothing I did brought my weight down. My obsession with the number on the scale came full circle, ending with Diana Schwarzbein's program.

Besides healing myself, I want to make sure that my ten-year-old daughter and my new baby daughter won't have their whole sense of worth centered around what they look like. If I can do anything, I'm going to make sure that my girls won't abuse themselves with food. I want to make sure that they never become focused on a number on the scale.

---

[1] *If you have unusual medical or nutritional needs or if you are pregnant or nursing, you should consult your physician.*

In order for this program to work, you must give up "dieting." As Elizabeth's story demonstrated, dieting, especially fasting, is the best way to destroy your metabolism. Any kind of nourishment-restrictive dieting will cause you to get fatter and fatter or thin and wasted.

The path to good health is often long. You cannot have a slender, healthy body overnight. The diet industry would like you to believe that, but it is a lie. The diet industry wants you to feel that you are an isolated, weak case and that people who do their programs correctly can achieve miraculous, overnight results. The truth is that the miracle comes when you return to the food chain and achieve nutritional and lifestyle balance. Once you are renourished, the "noise" in your head that demands that you eat an excess of carbohydrates and stimulants will go away. Quality of life is intrinsically bound to balanced nutrition.

Counting calories and fat grams and trying to "diet" by restricting calories and/or fat is destructive, emotionally and physically. More important, restricting nutrition will never get you to your goal of optimum health and ideal body composition. Stepping on the scale and looking for a particular number is destructive. With proper nourishment, your hormones and the neurotransmitters in your brain will regulate your food intake. By letting your body regulate the food you eat, you can throw away your bathroom scales. It does not matter what you weigh, it is body composition that counts.

When people hear the term "eating disorder," they think of anorexia or bulimia. But chronic dieting that leads to excessive body-fat gain, as in Elizabeth's case, is one form of eating disorder. Eating disorders take many forms and are not always obvious. But all imbalanced eating is destructive to your health. Sugar addiction is an eating disorder that causes many health problems, as you will learn in chapter 17.

Seventeen

Dr. Schwarzbein: Sugar Junkie

I have patients with health problems who ask me, "What did I do recently to get sick?" I tell them that it is not what they did just yesterday or the week before, the month before or even the year before. Problems do not arise overnight. Most disease does not appear suddenly. Body-fat gain, infertility and premature aging do not just happen. Nothing metabolic manifests itself overnight. Degenerative disease results from the cumulative poor eating and lifestyle habits you have had throughout your life. So recovery will not take place instantly, either. But your body can heal steadily.

I know because what I did to my body over the first eighteen years of my life destroyed my health. By changing my eating and lifestyle habits over the following nineteen years, I restored my health.

People say you cannot be too thin, but I was too thin as a child. In high school, my teachers thought I was anorexic. But I was not anorexic. I ate a lot of food. Unfortunately, most of it was junk.

I was a sugarholic. I would steal money from my parents to buy cotton candy, Pixie Sticks and Sweet Tarts. I did not like ice cream. I did not eat cake. I liked pure sugar. Things like white bread piled with sugar. My family is from Argentina and my mother used to make me *huevos con azúcar,* which is raw egg yokes with sugar mixed in, or buy me *dulce de leche,* which is caramelized milk sugar.

I was a picky eater otherwise. My mom would sit across the table from me at dinner and refuse to let me leave. Of course she had things to do, and I did not. Guess who could out-sit her mother every time?

In junior high I developed childhood asthma and chronic gastrointestinal problems. My mom asked doctors if eating too much sugar was causing my problems. Some doctors said, "It's not the sugar. Her problems are genetic." Others told her, "We think Diana's problems are in her head."

My mother always replied, "No, Diana is a very well-adjusted, happy child."

So I continued to eat as much sugar as I could.

I did well in school, even though I often stayed home sick and watched Elvis Presley movies and ate candy.

Since I had skipped third grade, when I was approaching puberty all my classmates were a year older. As I watched the older girls developing I thought, "Oh, that will be me next year." But that never happened. Although I started my period, I did not develop breasts and hips; I always looked like a prepubertal girl.

I was a tomboy. I wore jeans and never wore makeup. Maybe that was one reason I did not get into dieting. But I did continue to binge on sugar.

When I was eighteen, I fell apart. I went to Argentina to spend the summer with my relatives and came back twenty pounds heavier—all around my midsection. Suddenly I was overweight, had facial hair and cystic acne.

One of my cousins said, "What happened to you? You're so ugly."

Everyone said that the stress of the trip to Argentina made me eat more. But I had not eaten more. Still, I had gone from underweight to being overweight in two short months. Even though I was not happy with my new weight, I still did not go on a diet.

I returned to college that fall. I started noticing that without exercise, I felt anxious and buzzed all the time. Since I loved to run and swim and exercise, I took as many classes in P.E. as I could fit into my schedule. Even with all the exercise I could not get back to my previous low body-fat composition.

I started to read Adele Davis and took chemistry and biology courses. I realized for the first time that sugar was unhealthy. I thought, *Well, no wonder I have been so sick.* I thought it all out. Coke was bad; 7-Up was good. White sugar was bad, honey was good. It was a start, but of course later I learned that all sugar was the same.

I loved milk and drank it all day long until I was diagnosed with a lactose intolerance, which is the inability to digest milk sugar. So I used a milk substitute instead. I read cereal boxes to find those that contained no added sugar. For breakfast I ate shredded wheat with an eighth of a jar of honey and Mocha Mix instead of milk. I did not understand then that honey was just another form of sugar, nor did I know that Mocha Mix was filled with chemicals and damaged fats. I thought I was finally eating healthier foods because eliminating milk made me feel so much better. I did not realize that milk contained a lot of sugar.

But by the time I was nineteen years old, all food made me feel ill. I felt sick to my stomach constantly. It was a terrible cycle. If I did not eat, I felt sick from not eating; if I ate, I still felt sick. I thought I must be allergic to most foods.

I started going to the health food store. I ate "healthier" foods, such as granola with honey, but my asthma, intestinal problems and acne worsened. Doctors suspected ulcerative colitis or Crohn's disease. I got upper and lower intestinal X rays. I had a biopsy because they thought I might have sprue. But the tests all came back negative. More doctors insinuated that my illnesses were in my head. I was beginning to believe it. Others did not have answers. As a result, I was tagged with "irritable bowel syndrome."

Finally, in my fourth year of college, an endocrinologist told me, "Eat bland foods." After that, I ate anything I could find in the health food store that was bland. I started getting pegged as the woman who ate "cardboard food."

It was a constant battle to stay away from sugar. I had so much "noise" in my head. I craved all the food that made me sick, and the "noise" demanded I have it. I would eventually break down and eat candy bars and drink vanilla milkshakes, even though I was lactose intolerant. Afterward I was miserable.

During medical school I introduced vegetables and avocados back into my diet. I watched my progress objectively as I began to tolerate foods that I could not eat before. I thought either my illnesses were in my mind, or maybe I was getting over my food allergies.

By my mid-twenties, I was eating more proteins and fats and avoiding obvious sugar. I knew certain foods made me feel bad and others did not. Gradually as my diet improved the "noise" in my head went away and I no longer craved those foods that made me ill.

By age twenty-eight, my diet had improved to include a variety of foods, and by now I excluded most sugar from my diet. I was the healthiest I had ever been. I had lost body fat. My acne and facial hair disappeared. Even during my residency, when I was working long hours and staying up all night, I felt great.

I moved to Santa Barbara at age thirty and started to build a practice. My activity level drastically changed. When I was at Los Angeles County Hospital I had walked up and down eighteen flights of stairs to and from my office. Now in Santa Barbara I walked only up to the third floor and sat all day behind a desk.

From ages eighteen through thirty, I had proportionately decreased my sugar consumption, while increasing my exercise level. In so doing, I had developed a lean and fairly muscular body. But now, as I started getting fat on my thighs and around the middle, I thought it must be true what they say about turning thirty! I felt out of shape. I felt tired. I thought it was because I was sitting all the time and working twelve-hour days.

Although I was making better food choices, I was still eating more carbohydrates than my metabolism needed.

I reduced my carbohydrate consumption to match my current metabolism and activity level. I became stronger and felt better. I continued to watch my body recover from all the years of sugar abuse. I completely stopped having stomachaches, asthma and acne. At thirty-nine, I am the healthiest I have ever been in my life.

I understand now that my asthma, acne, delayed puberty and irritable bowel syndrome all stemmed from my high sugar consumption. I did not have genetic problems, food allergies or psychological difficulties. I had acquired insulin resistance and chronic conditions as a result of my eighteen years of sugar addiction. Because the conditions I suffered from were not genetic, I was able to reverse them with healthy eating and lifestyle changes.

Delayed Puberty

The purpose of puberty is to develop a fully functional hormone system that will change you from a child into an adult who can eventually procreate. Until you finish puberty, you do not develop an adult brain, and you do not develop a strong immune system. When you begin puberty, you have very low hormone systems. By the final stage of puberty, you will have fully developed hormone systems. After this system is developed, your eating and lifestyle habits will determine how healthy this system remains throughout your lifetime.

When you enter into puberty, sex hormone production begins and sets off communications between various body systems. If puberty is disrupted before a hormone system is fully developed, your body is left in a precarious situation. Since hormones are the communicators in your system, there is no coordination in the systems of your body. One imbalance creates another imbalance, because all the systems of the body are interconnected.

If a girl eats too much sugar, as I did, the resulting high insulin levels stimulate excess androgen production, which in turn blocks estrogen. This is a serious problem during puberty because the steady rise of estrogen levels and the subsequent actions of estrogen are needed to take a girl through the stages of puberty. This lack of estrogen rise results in delayed puberty. Also, without estrogen to balance out the androgens that are developed during puberty, you can develop acne.

Acne

Acne results from the clogging and subsequent inflammation of oil glands. When androgen activity increases, the number and secretion of the oil glands of the body also increase. The higher the secretion of oil, the more likely it is that oil glands will become clogged, resulting in acne.

Puberty and perimenopause are the two time periods when androgen activity increases. It used to be these times when women would complain of acne. Men generally experience acne only during puberty. But both women and men of all ages now complain of acne. The reason is that women and men are eating low-fat diets that are high in carbohydrates while also consuming stimulants. High carbohydrate consumption stimulates insulin production, and when insulin rises, androgens are increased beyond "normal" ranges. Stimulants exacerbate this while increasing insulin and adrenaline. It is true that sugar and chocolate can make you break out!

But acne is only one of the conditions I suffered from as a result of delayed puberty. Another problem was asthma.

Asthma

My high-sugar diet caused me to suffer from asthma, a condition marked by recurrent attacks of wheezing, or the inability to maintain adequate air flow.

Eating too many carbohydrates causes insulin levels to rise too high, which leads to the excess formation of hormones known as the eicosanoids. One of the eicosanoids' main functions is the relaxing or contracting of various smooth-muscle groups. Eicosanoids are also involved with immune-system responses. When insulin is high, it disrupts eicosanoid balance so that bronchial smooth muscles contract and immune responses are exaggerated. The end result is asthma.

There is a medical term, known as the Respiratory Quotient (RQ), that represents the amount of energy expended by the lungs to rid the body of the carbon dioxide generated by the metabolism of foods. Different foods have different RQs. The higher the RQ, the harder the lungs work. Carbohydrates have a quotient of 1; fats are much less at 0.7; and proteins come in at 0.9. Therefore, if you have asthma, your lungs will have to work even harder if you consume a lot of carbohydrates.

Another condition of my sugar addiction was irritable bowel syndrome.

Irritable Bowel Syndrome and Gluten Sensitivity

Irritable bowel syndrome is a term for any irritation of the bowel that cannot otherwise be categorized as a defined intestinal disease. Symptoms include intestinal bloating, gas pains, constipation and/or loose bowel movements.

To be absorbed, carbohydrates need to be digested in the small intestine into simple sugars. If you overeat carbohydrates, some of them will escape being digested into simple sugars and will continue on into the large intestine. Once carbohydrates enter the large intestine, the bacteria there will break down all the sugar into gas, which causes distention and pain. To make you feel even worse, water is pulled from the bloodstream into the colon to respond to the large sugar load that should not be there, resulting in loose stool.

Overconsuming carbohydrates can also cause gluten sensitivity, which I experienced. Gluten is found in whole-grain products and is used as a filler in many other products. Overconsuming gluten has caused an epidemic of gluten intolerance and hypersensitivity known as nontropical sprue. When you overeat gluten, your intestinal lining swells. This swelling prevents nutrients from being properly absorbed into your system, which leads to extreme B-vitamin deficiencies. Nontropical sprue has symptoms ranging from low energy, joint aches and pains, anemia, weight loss, edema and skin disorders, to diarrhea, abdominal discomfort and distention. Reducing your consumption of carbohydrates containing gluten and increasing your consumption of foods that contain B vitamins usually solves the problem.

Low Estrogen = Carbohydrate Craving

I have had women patients who could not stay on the healing program. They complained, "I can't do it." They told me they could not resist sugar and other stimulants.

I knew that women had the hardest time resisting sugar and other stimulants right before their periods, when estrogen is its lowest in the menstrual cycle. When I began to treat women with hormone replacement therapy they reported back to me that they had a much easier time resisting sugar. I learned then that low-estrogen states made it impossible for women to avoid carbohydrate craving, because estrogen is one of the hormones necessary for serotonin production. I now understand that even if at age eighteen I had known what I know now, with my hormone imbalances I could not have simply quit eating sugar. I was able to quit eating sugar over time, however, because several factors worked in my favor. First of all, I was young when I started to reverse my poor eating habits. Second, I had never dieted and so I did not have to reverse the damage that dieting does. Last of all, when I started eating protein and fat, my body was able to convert them into adequate estrogen. If I had waited until I was older and my sex-hormone production was declining (naturally, due to aging), then diet alone would not have been enough. I would have had to take hormone replacement therapy to achieve optimum health and my ideal body composition.

All stimulants—including stress—block estrogen action, which lowers serotonin levels, which leads to stimulant consumption, which leads to lower serotonin levels and so on. But if you eat properly and take hormone replacement therapy, if needed, your body will correct your low-estrogen state and your brain will produce serotonin, and your carbohydrate and stimulant cravings will vanish. But the only way to get over a low-estrogen state is to get through the healing process—and it takes time.

Sugar Addiction

Sugar interferes with the use of nutrients and damages your metabolism on a cellular level. Various real and man-made sugars are: sucrose (table sugar), fructose (fruit sugar), maltose (grain sugar), dextrose, polydextrose, corn syrup, molasses, sorbitol, maltodextrin and high-fructose corn syrup.

Since the low-fat movement has gained in popularity, many manufacturers have come out with low-fat food products sweetened with high-fructose corn syrup—the worst form of sugar. Many nutritional studies show that fructose ages your cells faster than sucrose.

Alcohol is another way to get sugar into your system. Alcohol is derived from grain or fruit, both of which are sugar.

Sugar addiction, whether due to various forms of refined sugar, man-made carbohydrates or alcohol, is an eating disorder. It took me awhile to accept that the term "eating disorder" had ever applied to me. Any addiction that takes away from balanced nutrition is indeed an eating disorder and can be cured by proper nutrition. My childhood sugar addiction caused me to suffer from acne, asthma and irritable bowel syndrome. Because I went through it, I understand the process of degeneration and the process of recovery.

I can now explain with biochemistry, physiology and endocrinology everything I have personally experienced. And I would not be able to understand how my patients feel if I had not experienced some of their symptoms myself. My own experience helps me to understand how impatient some people feel when they face what is sure to be a long road to recovery. When patients complain that the process takes too long, I remind them that it will take only a fraction of the years to build their bodies back up as it took to break their bodies down. It took me ten years to change my habits completely—but it would not have taken half that long if I had only known what I know now about nutrition and lifestyle.

While healing may seem to be a lengthy process, it is the only alternative if you want to get off the accelerated metabolic aging track. There is no reason to postpone good health. Each day that you eat a balanced diet, reduce stress, exercise and improve your lifestyle, you will feel better.

My sugar addiction started with a simple sweet tooth and became an irresistible and insatiable craving for sugar. However, some carbohydrate cravings begin with psychological trauma. Many people addicted to carbohydrates can trace their cravings back to a need for comfort and/or security. Vickie, in chapter 18, was traumatized as a young girl, and she turned to carbohydrates for comfort.

Eighteen

You *Can* Be Too Thin

Vickie was referred to me by her psychologist, who recognized that Vickie's problems, stemming from her past physical and psychological abuse, were exacerbated by her nutritionally imbalanced state. She was open about her anorexia and bulimia and eager to find a cure. Vickie was a tiny, frail-looking, thirty-four-year-old woman when she first came to see me.

Starving for the Answer

Vickie: When I think back on my life, my memories are associated with "food episodes." Each day of my life was a constant battle with food. I was a prisoner—obsessing about food, gorging myself on food, limiting food. Regrets. Guilt. Hating myself.

I grew up in a family where there was an unnatural focus on food. My father hoarded food. He had a vending business. He went to factories and places of business to supply the vending machines with cookies, cakes, candies, sodas, soups and coffee. The "inventory" was warehoused in our home. Tractor trailers made regular deliveries of food and filled the basement and garage.

When I was three, my mother was diagnosed with breast cancer and had a mastectomy. During my childhood, she had very serious operations related to her cancer.

My brother started sexually abusing me when I was little. I didn't tell on him because I was afraid, and also, in a weird way, I felt sorry for him when he begged me and said he was sorry.

With all these things going on in my family, it's no wonder that I started abusing myself with food at a very young age. I stuffed myself with cookies or cupcakes when I was upset or scared. I always ate in secret. Sugar was a drug. If I ate any sugar at all it led to wanting more and more. That first pleasurable taste would often send me into a frenzied state where I ate until I was sick. It was like a chemical reaction, demanding more and pushing me to eat extreme amounts.

I developed an internal list of good foods and bad foods. Food started to be on my mind all the time. I binged when I was nervous or upset. I shoved cookies into my mouth or took things into my room and ate them all really quickly. Whenever I binged, I purged with laxatives, exercise and fasting.

My mom and I used to bake cookies and cakes together. This started out to be a fun thing, but as I became obsessed with food, baking had a different purpose. I felt compelled to feed people all the things that I knew I shouldn't eat.

I became focused on how fat I thought I was. I stopped bingeing for awhile and began to deprive myself more and more. I ate smaller and smaller amounts of food. My parents were alarmed about my condition.

I exercised as much as I could. I always had my feet or something moving because I wanted to make sure that I was burning off calories. My parents wanted me to stop exercising. But I would go into the bathroom and turn on the shower to drown out the sound of my jumping jacks.

When I was thirteen, I was five feet, four inches and weighed seventy pounds. I was hospitalized. My anorexia was a cry for help.

During the next two years my mother's health declined and she was hospitalized quite a bit. She died when I was fifteen.

For the next several years, I either didn't eat enough or I binged—I'd make myself sick eating in a frenzied adrenaline state.

While I was eating I didn't care or even think about getting fat or about my health. But when I reached the point where I couldn't eat any more, the fears became overwhelming. I felt physically sick. I would cry and promise myself that I would never do it again. I felt desperate, scared and alone. I would look in the mirror and ask myself, "Who are you?"

I tried many times to throw up but couldn't. As the sugar wore off, I would crash. I had to have more sugar to calm down. The cycle would begin again.

During bingeing periods, I had stomachaches, my body ached and I felt hung over. All my organs hurt. I looked haggard. My body would be hot. I couldn't sleep. My hands and feet swelled and my face bloated. I got so bloated that someone once asked me if I was pregnant.

This cycle could go on for a few days to a few weeks. When it was all over, I was full of self-loathing. Semistarvation would begin. I would purge with laxatives, fasting and exercise. Or I would eat something like watermelon for several days. After that, I would go back to a strict low-fat, high-carb, low-calorie diet until my next binge. Mostly I was afraid of the next binge.

All through college my dad sent me "care" packages of vending-machine cookies and candy. Everyone thought that it was such a nice thing to do, but it created such a battle for me. I moved from the East Coast to Santa Barbara right after college to get away from all the old patterns, but my father's care packages followed me until I was in my thirties. I used to wish that it could be different with my dad, that he would come out to visit me and ask me what I really needed.

There was always a spirit in me to find something different. I spent all my time and all my money trying to get healthy. For years and years, I have been in therapy. Many therapists have wanted me to take antidepressants, or worse, they abandoned me as hopeless.

I always compared myself to others. I wanted to see what normal people ate. I was very curious. I would look at someone and wonder what that normal person consumed in a day. What choices did that normal person make?

I kept searching. I went to a nutritionist who put me on a high-carb diet. Oatmeal for breakfast with dates in it. Carrot juice, potatoes, yams, lentils. I felt crazy. I binged more and more. I was constantly hungry.

I met my husband Alex in 1991. I wasn't honest with him in the beginning. I didn't say, "I have an eating disorder." He heard "Am I fat?" questions. Or, "Oh, I ate so much." But once my anorexia started coming out and I started working more with my therapist, it frightened him.

Alex: I have always been attracted to thin women. I met Vickie at an emotional-growth seminar. She was thin and attractive. It was a long-distance, weekend relationship. A couple of times, she pointed out that she couldn't eat this or that. It just went over my head. I would visit her and she'd fix dinner for herself—a potato and vegetables. That's dinner? I didn't get it.

We got married after being involved for a year and a half. Then the pressure cooker started. I never witnessed a binge. She's very good at hiding. But she would tell me that she ate a few muffins, and really beat herself up about it. I would ask myself, why is she doing this? For me it was like she was abusing herself. I didn't get it. I'd hear about her eating disorder in the abstract, but that's not like being there to see a binge. I wasn't willing to accept her eating disorder. I took a hard-line position.

Vickie: I wanted to include Alex in my therapy. I told him what was going on. But he continued to get mad at me when I binged. He was frightened. His fear prevented him from being compassionate. So I stopped telling him if I binged. I was already beating myself up enough.

At one point, my therapist said, "Vickie, you have the understanding emotionally, and you've done so much work over the years. But I think there's something going on physiologically." She referred me to Diana Schwarzbein.

Dr. Schwarzbein got it right away. She said, "You're undernourished." She had me do a bone scan. The bone density in my hip was 26 percent below what the bones of someone thirty-four years old should be. Dr. Schwarzbein said, "Don't go skiing or anything like that right now." It was a shock to realize what I'd done to my body.

She understood what I had been through. She explained the physiology to me, described a new way to eat and what it was going to do for me. She told me how to eat. *What* to eat. She encouraged me to put fat in my diet.

I took a good look at myself. I didn't want to keep ruining my life. I didn't want to ruin my body anymore. I accepted what she said. It was such a relief.

Dr. Schwarzbein: When I first saw Vickie, she had limp, dull hair, a pasty complexion and no muscle tone. Her body looked like that of a prepubescent girl. She was in a desperate state, physically and emotionally. Vickie was suffering from anorexia nervosa and bulimia. Anorexia nervosa used to occur mainly in females between the ages of twelve and twenty-one. Now we are seeing anorexia in all ages, and in men as well as women. Anorexics have an intense fear of fat. Even though they may starve themselves and exercise to the point of emaciation, this fear does not go away. The anorexic, no matter how thin, always "feels fat."

Bulimia is a disorder of excessive and insatiable appetite. Bulimics binge-eat and then induce vomiting and/or diarrhea with a dangerous use of laxatives. They may follow a binge with extreme exercise, strict dieting or fasting. Bulimics, like anorexics, have an exaggerated concern about their body shape and weight. It is possible to suffer, like Vickie, from both conditions.

Both anorexia and bulimia are caused by undernourishment and neurotransmitter imbalances. They are not genetic diseases but are acquired when a person becomes emotionally and physically ill.

When I explained how the healing program could help her, I emphasized that she would not get fat but that she would gain pounds as she filled out her hollow bones and her muscle mass. I explained that it was normal to have a protective layer of fat under the skin, but, again, this did not mean she would be getting fat rolls. Instead of her old goal of weighing as little as possible, her new goal would be to allow her body to reach its ideal composition. She would be heavier on the scale—but she would still be slender since this extra weight would be mostly bone and lean muscle mass.

"Noise"

In addition to her intense fear of fat, the "noise" in Vickie's head demanded that she binge on carbohydrates to increase the release of serotonin. Between binges, Vickie adhered to a strict diet that was low-calorie, low-fat and high-carbohydrate. This diet actually triggered bingeing episodes by lowering serotonin and turning up the volume of "noise" in Vickie's head. But, tracing it back farther, her serotonin levels had been low for a very long time, beginning with the stress of her early emotional traumas. Again, stress depletes serotonin.

Vickie constantly thought about sugar because the brain cries out for carbohydrates when there is no ongoing serotonin production. As you learned in chapter 4, this "noise" causes stimulant craving as well. I use carbohydrate or stimulant cravings as an indicator of metabolic health. *If you crave any form of stimulants, carbohydrates or otherwise, then you are not healthy.* If you crave carbohydrates or stimulants, your serotonin levels are low. Your brain demands stimulants to raise your serotonin levels.

Vickie's stimulant of choice was carbohydrates. Her bingeing on carbohydrates led to all the symptoms of reactive hypoglycemia, or low blood sugar. Although hypoglycemia means low blood sugar, your blood sugar levels never drop below normal ranges. What you are actually experiencing is the side effect of the rising adrenaline levels. The symptoms of hypoglycemia are nausea, shakiness, clamminess, sweating, lightheadedness, irritability, racing heart, anxiety and carbohydrate craving (not necessarily all symptoms at the same time).

Reactive hypoglycemia occurs when you eat too many carbohydrates at one time. This increases insulin levels, which alerts the liver that too much sugar might reach the brain. In order to protect the brain, insulin diverts that sugar to fat production. However, when this happens your brain is not getting enough sugar, so adrenaline is released from the adrenal gland, making the liver release sugar into the bloodstream to maintain tightly regulated amounts of sugar going to the brain. At the same time, your brain demands that you eat more carbohydrates. This in turn releases even more insulin, which again alerts the liver. The liver then diverts most of that sugar to fat production. This is why eating carbohydrates is only a temporary solution to reactive hypoglycemia.

In Vickie's case, both her reactive hypoglycemia and low-serotonin state kept her bingeing until she was physically unable to eat another bite.

Elizabeth, Vickie and I are all examples of people with eating disorders. Eating disorders take many forms but are always destructive to physical and emotional health. There is no question that eating disorders are epidemic in our culture. Once a person enters into a destructive eating pattern, whether it is a sugar addiction, bingeing or starving, the "noise" in that person's head is often so loud and so constant that he or she typically cannot hear the voice of reason. I have found that when a patient satisfies the body's need for proper nutrition and hormone balances, the "noise" goes away. The patient is then on his or her way to complete recovery, which includes reaching an ideal body composition.

Osteoporosis

Before I explained anything to Vickie, I gave her the results of her bone-density test. She was shocked to see that she had the bones of a seventy-year-old woman. I told her that her greatest health threat was osteoporosis. This was a very real danger, as osteoporosis claims more lives per year than breast cancer.

Many women, like Vickie, do not understand the grave danger of being too thin. Eating a low-fat, high-carbohydrate diet or a low-calorie diet results in no muscle tone and hollow bones. That is why Vickie weighed very little on the scale. Like Vickie, many women focus only on the number on the scale and do not realize the repercussions of maintaining a low body weight.

Normal Bone Formation

In order to understand osteoporosis, you must first understand how healthy bones are formed. Bones are tissues that are constantly remodeling. They need to break down and rebuild themselves in order to maintain structural integrity. Contrary to popular belief, bones are not just calcium. Think of bones as tubes that are made of, and filled with, protein and hardened by calcium. The hardening of this protein is what makes bone solid.

The body contains specialized cells for breaking down and forming bone. The *osteoclast* cells break down and eliminate old bone. The *osteoblast* cells lay down new bone matrix, which is made up of collagen. Collagen, a protein, is the "backbone" of bone. After the bone matrix is laid down, hormones direct calcium to be laid down on top of the protein. This new bone matrix is now calcified. This calcified bone matrix is mature bone.

Osteoclast and osteoblast (breakdown and buildup) functions are coupled with and modulated by many hormones. For example, estrogen slows down the activity of the osteoclast cells, thereby slowing the breakdown process of bone remodeling. Progesterone and androgens (testosterone, DHEA) stimulate the formation of new bone through the osteoblasts.

In prepuberty, your bones are just beginning to fill in with collagen. When your sex hormones turn on, the collagen is calcified, which results in more solid, heavier bones. Throughout your teen years, bones continue to fill in as a result of good nutrition, normal hormone development and the passage of time. If your bones become denser, your weight must go up. No one tells girls or young women that they are supposed to weigh more every decade as their hollow bones fill up. Teenage girls who do not understand that they should weigh more begin to diet to lose the few extra pounds they have gained on the scale. Too often, those few extra pounds are bones. If you continue to try to stay the same weight and maintain the sizes you wore as a teenager, you will not build enough bone mass.

Because peak bone mass correlates with peak sex-hormone production, bone mass peaks between the ages of twenty and thirty. Calcified, solid bones weigh much more than hollow bones, and these calcified, solid bones signify a strong and healthy body. Keeping up this peak bone-mass level is directly related to the aging process. When sex-hormone production goes down, you begin to lose bone mass. In other words, aging is a natural process involving the loss of hormones, and therefore bone loss is a natural result. At age ninety, a healthy woman who has not been on any hormone replacement therapy would be expected to have less bone mass than in her peak bone-mass years.

When Bone Formation Is Disrupted

Disruption of normal bone metabolism leads to less bone formation and/or increased bone breakdown. Both these processes lead to osteopenia (less bone). When this decreased bone mass leads to fracture, we call this disease osteoporosis. Osteopenia does not always lead to osteoporosis. For example, children have less bone mass, or osteopenia, but they do not have osteoporosis. If you have not reached your peak bone mass by age twenty to thirty this is osteopenia, but not necessarily osteoporosis. However, less peak bone mass after the age of thirty puts you at a higher risk for osteoporosis later in life.

Osteopenia is on the rise in younger women for two reasons: First, like Vickie, some women are so afraid of gaining weight that they deprive their bodies of proteins and fats, so they never reach peak sex-hormone levels; thus they never develop good peak bone-mass. Their bodies use their potential bone protein stores for immediate survival. Often these same women use caffeine to curb their appetites. Caffeine and other stimulants are known to cause bone loss.

Other women believe low-fat claims and cut back on proteins and fats while increasing exercise, in an attempt to avoid heart disease or breast cancer. Even though they reached a good peak bone mass in their twenties, they then begin to lose bone rapidly from poor eating habits. Bone thinning occurs on low-fat, low-protein and/or low-calorie diets because protein deprivation leads to both decreased collagen formation and increased collagen utilization by the body.

Exercising without feeding your body enough food from the four nutrient groups will accelerate bone loss, since the body is forced to use even more of your own structural proteins.

Current popular belief is that taking in enough calcium and getting enough exercise can prevent the loss of bone. If only it were that easy. You need protein, calcium and balanced hormones for bone production. Every day I explain to another woman that calcium pills and exercise are not the answer to osteoporosis prevention. I explain that proteins and fats are essential nutrients for bone formation. Protein is necessary for bone collagen, and fats are required for sex-hormone production, which fosters healthy bones.

Exercise increases bone production when you eat enough proteins and fats so that new bone can be formed. When you do not eat enough proteins and fats, exercise actually accelerates bone loss.

But this is not the only way that exercise can damage your bones. Overexercising causes insulin and sex-hormone levels to drop. This is apparent in long-distance runners and other women who overtrain. Any behavior that results in low insulin levels and low sex hormones will cause rapid bone loss.

Women with low bone mass (osteopenia) are at greater risk for developing osteoporosis. However, a low bone-density reading in a young woman and a low bone-density reading in a old woman have two different meanings. If you do not reach a good peak bone mass or if you destroy your peak bone mass with poor eating and lifestyle habits, you are putting yourself at a higher risk for osteoporosis when you are older. If you are past menopause and you have decreased bone mass, you may already have osteoporosis and be at an immediate risk for fracturing.

There are two types of osteoporosis. Senile osteoporosis is due to the gradual loss of hormones seen in normal aging. Menopausal osteoporosis is due to accelerated hormone losses seen around menopause. Both can be accelerated by a low-fat, low-protein and/or low-calorie diet, increased stimulant use, and anything that decreases insulin below normal levels.

Two areas of excessive bone fractures seen in patients with either type of osteoporosis are the spine and hip. Spinal compression fractures result in small vertebral breaks that gradually collapse the spine. This spinal collapse, if it occurs in the upper spine, is referred to as a "dowager's hump." Quality of life is significantly decreased in a woman with compression fractures of the spine. This can be a very painful phenomenon and extremely difficult to treat. Some afflicted women get hooked on pain pills and/or are wheelchair-bound. Women with osteoporosis also have a greater potential for long bone fractures. An elderly woman with a fractured hip bone has a 50 percent chance of dying in the next year due to a blood clot in the lungs. This occurs because mobility is restricted in older individuals. Less active older women are more apt to develop blood clots because of blood pooling in one area, and from lower estrogen levels.

The Prevention
and Treatment of Osteoporosis

Taking calcium and exercising are not ways to prevent osteoporosis. To prevent osteoporosis you need to achieve and maintain good healthy peak bone mass. To do this, you should:

- Eat a well-balanced diet including calcium-rich foods: almonds, asparagus, brewer's yeast, broccoli, cabbage, dairy foods, dandelion greens, dulse, filberts, green leafy vegetables, kale, kelp, mustard greens, oats, parsley, salmon (with bones), sardines, seafood, sesame seeds, tofu and turnip greens.

- Exercise according to your food intake.

- Do not use stimulants: alcohol, amphetamines, Armour thyroid, caffeine, chocolate, cocaine and other "recreational" drugs, dextroamphetamine sulfate (Dexedrine), diet pills, ma huang, methylphenidate hydrochloride (Ritalin), over-the-counter cold medications, phentermine (the phen in Phen Fen), sugar, tobacco or excess triiodothyronine (Cytomel, the active thyroid hormone).

• Avoid anti-inflammatory drugs as much as possible: aspirin, ibuprofen and all the nonsteroidal anti-inflammatory drugs, and steroids such as prednisone.

• Do not take medication that stops your menstrual cycle.

• Alert your physician, to find out the cause, if you skip more than three periods or have irregular periods.

• Take hormone replacement therapy in menopause.

It is never too late to reverse bone loss. Even if you have inadvertently destroyed bone mass, the above seven steps will help reverse the damage that has been done. Furthermore, women who have osteoporosis have been told that this condition is irreversible; however, this is not true. Even if you have documented osteoporosis with a fracture, the above lifestyle changes will help your body form new healthy bone regardless of your age.

> **Vickie:** I still binged a lot in the beginning. Dr. Schwarzbein guided me, encouraged me, made sense of the stages I was going through. She even said that if I had to binge, I should eat something that has fat in it, like real ice cream.
>
> I wasn't as upset after I binged. I knew that I was on the right path to getting better. Instead of my bingeing episodes lasting days or weeks, a binge would go for one day, then a half a day, then an hour.
>
> I've kept food journals ever since I first saw Dr. Schwarzbein two years ago. I wanted to understand whether I was eating a lot of food or not enough. If I did binge, we could look back and check out what I had eaten a couple of days before, or see if maybe I wasn't getting enough fats. I've learned to stay away from Chinese food or anything that has hidden sugars in it because I'm so sensitive to sugar. Even if little bits of sugar crept in, I would start carbo-craving.

Dr. Schwarzbein had me put essential oils into my diet. She asked me to eat avocados. The idea of eating foods that I thought were high in calories scared me to death. But then I began to understand—the fat kept me satiated so I wasn't hungry or craving carbs anymore.

I've had definite ups and downs. But my life is dramatically changed. As I began to get nourished, my depression lifted. All of a sudden, I could think and have creative thoughts. The real me is emerging! The psychological and the physiological are intertwined. It's amazing to me that I can live life and not think about eating. My self-esteem has increased. At thirty-six years old, I finally feel like an adult who can express opinions and not worry about making waves or pleasing everyone. I feel balanced emotionally. I have more energy, more muscle and more endurance. My hair has gotten shiny and my coloring is much more vibrant. I feel pretty for the first time.

Dry, Thinning Hair, Wrinkles and Cellulite

Hair is a tissue made up of keratin that constantly replaces itself by falling out and growing back. But hair loss occurs when the growth process is slowed or ceases. To make hair, you need protein, fats, a good blood supply to the scalp and normal hormone levels. When you do not eat sufficient proteins and fats to keep up the ongoing replenishment of your body, it is forced to use its own resources. When your body uses its own proteins for survival, structural proteins (bones, hair, muscles, nails) are always sacrificed before functional proteins (enzymes, hormones, neurotransmitters). Of course, this type of hair loss is not the same as baldness, which is for the most part genetic and not reversible.

Anemia reduces blood flow to the scalp, and we know that low-fat, low-protein diets can cause anemia. Too many carbohydrates and stress (including the stress of starvation) increase the levels of the hormones cortisol and testosterone to above normal. Both high cortisol and testosterone levels cause hair loss. Last but not least, when your body is starving, all metabolic processes slow down. Low-fat diets cause low-thyroid activity as a protection mechanism to save energy, which translates to hair loss.

The good news is that hair loss caused by protein and fat deficiencies is completely reversible with balanced nutrition and/or hormone replacement therapy.

In addition to dry, thin hair, you will see dry skin, wrinkles and prematurely aged faces on the people who eat low-fat diets. This is because you need protein to make up the tissues of the skin, hormones (derived from cholesterol) to keep the skin plump (hydrated) and oils to keep the skin lubricated.

Another symptom of chronic dieting is cellulite. Cellulite—fatty, lumpy deposits under the skin—accumulates as the result of dieting or from eating an imbalanced diet. Since women have more estrogens than androgens, their fat deposits are stored around the hips and thighs. To get rid of cellulite you must stop dieting and go on the healing program, which will increase your metabolism and your muscle mass.

Vickie: I began to get stronger, and it was apparent to Alex. When I got more opinionated and assertive, Alex understood that I was getting healthier.

I eat like a normal person now, a lot of food and more consistently. Real meals. I'll have a big breakfast, then I'll have a big lunch, and I don't even think about it. Being nourished and having correct proportions of protein, fat and carbohydrates leaves me feeling satisfied, so I don't need to constantly think about food like I used to. I order what I want in a restaurant, within the framework of the program. Before, it was always whatever was the least fat, the least calories. Now it's the opposite.

I didn't put on a lot of weight eating this way. I thought I would, but I haven't. When I went to see Dr. Schwarzbein, I weighed 100 pounds. Now I weigh about 110. Learning about the healing program has changed my life. I never knew I could see life differently. I don't see a therapist now. I can buy clothes. I can live life, not think about food.

Alex and I are going to try to have a baby. Before, I was never stable enough emotionally or physically. It's a miracle. Just nourishing myself has made my life so different.

Dr. Schwarzbein: Although it was hard for Vickie to put fat in her diet, she did. She noticed immediately that it helped with some of the "noise" in her head.

After two years on the program, Vickie is a new woman. Her hair is shinier, her skin is more supple now. She has gained some lean body mass (bones and muscle). However, she is still underweight. Vickie needs to continue on the healing program to fill in her hollow bones and gain lean muscle mass.

Her outlook on life is improved. She is able to think clearly, enjoy life and her work. Vickie put a lot of effort into this program and still does. She understands that she cannot spend over twenty years destroying her metabolism and expect it to come back overnight. She has rough times and falls back on bingeing but she continues to stick it out. She is on the road to recovery.

Vickie's story demonstrates that the human body is extremely resilient and initially will seem to take a lot of abuse. Disease and chronic conditions do not happen overnight. The slow metabolic destruction involved with not eating correctly will, over time, lead to the accelerated metabolic aging process. On the outside you may look good. On the inside it is not pretty. You cannot starve your body without incurring a cost.

Vickie's childhood trauma resulted in an eating disorder that caused her to become too thin and malnourished. Chapter 19 tells the story of Alex, who suffered as a result of a lifetime of excesses.

Nineteen

Overfed and Undernourished

Many Americans have not adopted the low-fat lifestyle and are not protein deprived. We like ice cream, fast foods, soft drinks and beer. We rarely exercise. We weigh about thirty-five pounds too much on average and we are tired, suffering from chronic illnesses and conditions. We have accepted that aches and pains and physical ailments are a natural part of adulthood. But this is not true. The human body is capable of great strength, endurance and longevity, given proper nutrition.

Balanced nutrition is the key to good health. As you learned in chapter 3, humans cannot put just anything into their bodies with impunity. Saccharin, margarine, other invented substances, refined and processed foods, caffeine, alcohol, tobacco and aspartame are damaging to the human physiology. Advertising tries to convince us that these substances are healthy, wholesome and, if nothing else, gratifying. But these substances are toxins; they raise insulin levels, or imbalance other hormones, and they literally poison our bodies.

Remember the principle: *Degenerative diseases are not genetic but acquired. Because the systems of the human body are interconnected and because one imbalance creates another imbalance, poor eating and lifestyle habits, not genetics, cause degenerative disease.*

Because metabolism proceeds on a cellular level, we have to think about what we put into our bodies. When you put damaging substances into your body, the damage occurs out of sight. You travel along the accelerated metabolic aging track and your health deteriorates. When you begin to experience body-fat gain and health problems, these problems seem as if they occurred overnight.

When Alex, a thirty-nine-year-old professional man, gained body fat and had a health crisis, it seemed as if his problems developed suddenly. Alex came to me at his wife's urging. His wife, Vickie, whom you read about in the previous chapter, had experienced great success on the healing program. Though Alex had witnessed Vickie's recovery, he felt that he did not need to change his own diet and lifestyle habits.

Man of Extremes

Alex: I've had many addictions in my life that have taken a toll on my body. Growing up, my diet consisted of lots of protein—meat and cheese—lots of sugar and fat, like ice cream, Ding Dongs, Scooter Pies, candy, doughnuts and sodas, potatoes and crackers, and very few vegetables or fruits.

Most of my life I've been physically active. From fourteen to twenty I ran track and cross-country, averaging ten to fifteen miles a day. I always played baseball and basketball, skied, rode bikes and hiked. My self-image has always been that of an athlete. Contrary to this self-image, from fifteen to thirty-five, I smoked two to three packs of cigarettes a day. At about 150 pounds, I was always lean for my height, with a resting heart rate as low as thirty-eight and body fat of 6 percent.

My addictions started in my teens—beginning with smoking, relationships with girls and work. By the time I was eighteen, I was working in a small, high-tech corporate environment forty to forty-five hours a week, attending college, carrying nineteen units a semester and planning a wedding. I got married and bought my own home. That same year I was hospitalized for ten days with colitis. I went on to struggle with diarrhea for eighteen years.

At a very young age, I figured out that I was responsible for my own health. But I didn't really know how or what to do about it. I was always juggling a million things, and felt if I tried to stop everything I would crash. Within three and a half years my first marriage broke up, but I continued on the fast track. I was burned out from work and disillusioned with school, so I quit both.

I poured myself into a new job in the high-tech industry. It was a fast-growing company, and I was given unlimited opportunity. I traveled often and worked an average of eighty to a hundred hours per week for eight years. During that period I'd typically have a Danish for breakfast and three to six cups of coffee with two rounded spoons of sugar in each cup. I'd grab a late lunch of a deli sandwich. Later I'd put away a six-pack of Pepsi, several candy bars and a fast-food or restaurant dinner. I didn't smoke much in the morning, but by the afternoons and late nights I was a chimney. I averaged three to four hours of sleep a night, often staying up all night.

I never seemed to have any shortage of relationships. I wanted a family but was too afraid of screwing it up—or getting screwed. I also noticed how frequently I was ill. My heart rate, body fat and weight increased. I had to watch my weight for the first time in my life. I had typically eaten four meals a day plus snacks. This changed to three meals a day plus snacks. I reduced my protein and ate a lot more carbs—after all, carbs were supposed to be good "energy" food.

I began therapy, reduced my work to forty-five to fifty-five hours per week, quit smoking and reached out to make friends. I worked with a gastroenterologist to clean up my digestive problems. I started getting six-and-a-half to eight hours of sleep a night and slowed down my relationships with women.

After a year or two I met Vickie, who would become my second wife. When I was thirty-five everything in my life changed—I moved, changed jobs and got married. It felt like the best year of my life. But things didn't stay as good.

The city I moved to, to join my wife, is noted for its beauty. But I found it difficult adjusting to my new home. I took up golf to make new friends. On New Year's Day in 1995, I tore my knee while practicing at the driving range. The pain of the injury triggered headaches.

At that time, my wife was a patient of Dr. Schwarzbein's and was showing noticeable results on the eating program. She was always after me to do it, too. I'd say, "I eat the same things you fix. So what if I cheat a little?" I thought my diet was good. But the headaches kept getting worse. I'd wake up in the middle of the night, with night sweats and a clenched jaw. I started feeling depressed because my life had changed so much. I had always been athletic and active, but it felt like everything had changed overnight.

I finally went to see Dr. Schwarzbein and she explained the eating program, but I wasn't ready for it.

Next I saw a neurologist who diagnosed me with migraines and gave me four different types of medication. The plan was to build up the levels of these "preventive" medications in my system to reverse the cycle of headaches and then, hopefully, eliminate the nightly medications over time. The frequency of my headaches reduced dramatically over a period of six months, but the combination of the different medications had an adverse effect on my digestive system.

I had suffered terrible intestinal problems my entire adult life. Now these problems were compounded. I was miserable a lot and even had to go to the emergency room several times because of severe abdominal pain. I didn't sleep well. I had night sweats to the point where we were changing the sheets every night. I was lethargic in the morning. Things had gotten so bad I began to wonder if I would end up with a colostomy. It was not the kind of life I wanted. How much longer could I go through this?

Since my remarriage I thought I'd been eating much better. My typical breakfast was now a bowl of "healthy" cereal with fruit and Rice Dream ["milk" made from rice]. If I had meetings at work and couldn't get a mid-morning snack, I would start to get the shakes inside. My mind would just go someplace and I couldn't think about anything. I would excuse myself to eat some cheese and crackers, or I'd be a basket case with a migraine headache. After fifteen months of inactivity, migraine headaches and otherwise poor health, my weight went up to 185. I was very uncomfortable in my body.

At my wife's urging, I saw Dr. Schwarzbein again twelve months after our first meeting. She talked to me about the nutritional program again. This time I was receptive.

Dr. Schwarzbein: The first time Alex came to see me, he listened while I described my program of nutrition, stress reduction and exercise, but he was seeking a magic pill for his ailments. Unfortunately, there is no pill that can cure problems related to a lifestyle like Alex's. I understand how overwhelming it is for people to make significant lifestyle changes when they feel mentally and physically depleted. People like Alex often come back to me after hitting bottom. Alex finally realized he needed to take control of his own health. At the second meeting, he was ready to get serious about changing his lifestyle.

I explained that headaches occur in many forms and are caused by a variety of conditions. Some headaches are caused by poor nutrition, stress or overuse of stimulants. These types of headache stem from increases in the chemicals that cause pain. Low serotonin levels are responsible for overproduction of these chemicals, which then cause pain through inflammation, vasodilatation and smooth-muscle contraction. Re-establishing proper serotonin levels through nutrition and hormone balancing eliminates these types of headaches.

Alex also experienced fatigue. Fatigue can be brought on by various problems. One of these is poor sleeping or insomnia. Poor nutrition contributes to insomnia by causing serotonin depletion. (See chapter 4 for more on insomnia and low serotonin.)

Alex: I changed my regular breakfast to an omelet with butter, sautéed spinach and feta cheese, plus whole-grain toast with butter. Within two weeks, I no longer needed a morning snack for the first time in my memory. For lunch I generally have protein and two small servings of vegetables, like coleslaw or broccoli, and corn, peas or lima beans. For dinner I have a healthy serving of chicken or fish, occasionally red meat, and a good-sized serving of two different vegetables.

I sleep all night without getting up for the bathroom. I rarely sweat at night. I'm no longer lethargic in the morning. I'm up out of bed and into work early. I'm a different person. Before, I had twenty severe migraines a month; now I'm down to three or four a month, with much less severity. I'm beginning to understand how critical proper nutrition is to avoid migraines.

During the first eight weeks on the program, I lost fifteen pounds naturally and didn't feel at all food deprived.

Recently my knee injury was diagnosed as requiring surgery. Since the surgery, I've been in an aggressive physical rehab program. It feels great being active.

I've mellowed out in my life, particularly over the past six years. I'm much more aware of the choices that I make and the consequences of those choices on my life. I still have some bad habits and can be that "man of extremes." But I don't feel this diet is an extreme program. I am stronger and feel more stability in my life. As I look into the future, I feel inspired and excited. Both my wife and I are maintaining a healthier lifestyle through balanced nutrition. We're looking forward to having a child now. I am planning to play with my kids and retain the physique of an athlete into my retirement years.

Dr. Schwarzbein: Alex had gone through years of abusing his own body. The miracle is that the human body is truly regenerative. Alex's story is just one of many where a few crucial changes resulted in dramatic improvement.

We would all like to spare our children the suffering that results from a lifetime of excess. The question is how? Chapter 20 will examine what happens to children who eat an imbalanced diet and what you can do about it.

Twenty

Children Do Not
Have to Be Overweight

In the last twenty years, we have gotten farther away from the food chain by feeding our kids processed food products. Many processed foods have at least some of the fat removed. These products are then filled with either chemicals or more sugar to give them flavor. Processed foods are fattening, first, because they contain sugar, which raises insulin levels and, second, because they instigate the vicious cycle of carbohydrate craving. This is why many children are overweight today. To make matters worse, children now eat low-fat foods. Unfortunately, we have been taught to worry more about the fat content than the chemical and sugar content of these foods. We have been led to believe that, as long as there is little or no fat, we are doing no harm. Soon if other fat-replacement chemical compounds, such as the already approved Olestra, are allowed by the FDA, processed foods will contain no real, healthy fat at all.

Adults need fat in their diet to replenish and nourish the body, but children need fat even more to develop into healthy adults. Fatty foods are the source of the fat-soluble vitamins A, E, D and K. Taking vitamin supplements has not shown the same health benefits as eating the fatty foods that contain these fat-soluble vitamins.

Children go through many stages as they mature toward adulthood. All of these stages require proper nourishment. During these stages when hormones are turning on, children will gain body fat if they eat incorrectly. When some parents see the first sign of this fat gain, they panic, jump to the wrong conclusions and put their children on "weight-loss" programs. These weight-loss programs are destructive to children's health and do nothing to reduce body fat. In fact, the first "diet" often propels the child into a lifetime of yo-yo dieting.

What parents do not realize is that children are not doing anything different. They have always eaten the same way! But the hormone changes that begin in puberty expose poor nutrition for what it really is. Instead of recognizing that poor eating habits are the source of weight gain, parents blame the child for overeating.

Let me explain how hormone changes can affect your child's weight. Even though many hormone changes occur during puberty, we will focus only on the androgen hormone changes and their effect on insulin and fat gain.

The first stage of puberty is adrenarche (when the adrenal gland turns on). At this time both boys and girls start to produce androgens. If, during this stage of puberty, a child is eating poorly, the resulting high insulin levels stimulate even higher levels of androgens. High androgens plus high insulin levels produce abnormal body-fat gain, especially around the midsection. With this weight gain, the child and parents may panic. Parents say, "You need to go on a diet. You're eating too many calories. Let's cut down on fats."

So the child goes on a low-fat, high-carbohydrate diet and continues to gain body fat. I have had children tell me that they have stuck faithfully to their diet. They eat cereal and fruit for breakfast, and pasta and other starches for lunch and dinner. They are hungry all the time. What is worse, with the inevitable body-fat gain from this diet, their parents accuse them of cheating. I have even seen cases where parents have gone as far as taking their children to "obesity specialists," who have diagnosed their problems as genetic. This is a tragedy.

When children come to me for "genetic obesity," I immediately switch them to a balanced diet sufficient in proteins and fats while decreasing their carbohydrate consumption. Every one of these children loses body fat and gains her or his ideal body composition.

Children who remain on a low-fat, high-carbohydrate diet have in store a lifetime of heartache and disease. Children's insulin levels rise from the same stimuli that raise adult insulin levels. Before puberty, however, because children do not have fully developed hormone systems, you do not see the problems that can occur from high insulin levels. During puberty more hormone systems turn on. Because all the systems of the body are interconnected, one imbalance creates another imbalance.

You read about Elizabeth, who was pushed into low-calorie dieting as a young girl. Her early attempts at weight loss through depriving her body of nourishment led to devastating results that continued throughout her adult life. The trend is even worse today. These days, a low-fat diet is the popular "weight-loss" method for children. But as you have learned, low-fat dieting is more harmful to your children's health and development than low-calorie dieting. Marilyn, a sixty-five-year-old woman, had a childhood experience with weight gain that will serve as a valuable lesson for many parents.

> **Marilyn:** When I was fifteen years old, in 1946, people weren't thin like they are now. In those days, we had a store called The House of Nine for the teeniest girls, who wore a size nine—that was considered very little back then. My mother was considered a beautiful woman and she wore a size sixteen. Even young girls wore girdles. Because if your stomach stuck out or your bottom wobbled or whatever, you didn't want that—there was a certain look, and girdles were just part and parcel of that look.
>
> People weren't dieting as much at that time, either. In fact, I was coming home from school every day and eating cookies, milk and cake. I was eating up a storm. One day in science class the teacher asked, "Who in this class eats a good breakfast in the morning?" I was eating waffles and pancakes every morning, so I raised my hand. I was the only person in

the class who raised my hand. The teacher looked at me and said, "Boys and girls, I want you to take a good look at Marilyn. Look at how rosy her cheeks are. She's the only one who looks like she's eaten a good breakfast." I thought that was fine at the time.

Two weeks later I was walking down the hall at school, and I caught a reflection of myself in a windowpane. Those were the days when we wore angora sweaters. I was wearing a yellow angora sweater with long fluffy fur. I had long, very blond hair, and with the angora sweater I looked like a giant Easter bunny just moving right along there. I really hadn't noticed myself before because the weight gain had happened so gradually. But now I ran to the pay phone at lunchtime and called my mother. I said, "Mom, you have to make an appointment for me with the doctor." She took me to the doctor very willingly. Not one word about my weight—I was five feet, six inches and weighed 143 pounds. I guess she was smart enough to keep silent.

The doctor was a Swedish man. He put me on a protein diet. I had eggs in the morning with a piece of toast. For lunch I had a chicken breast, lots of raw vegetables and maybe a hard-boiled egg. My mother used to buy pineapple spears at the farmer's market, and that's what I had for dessert. Dinner was salad with oil and vinegar dressing, a big piece of meat and vegetables. On Sundays I ate whatever I wanted to. Still I went from 143 to 129 pounds—fourteen pounds in two months.

There have been times in my life when I didn't eat properly and gained a few pounds. But I can honestly say that I have never had a weight problem again. My diet is not skimpy. As a matter of fact, I do eat quite a bit of food. I just make sure it's the right food.

Dr. Schwarzbein: Marilyn's story illustrates the fact that at one time people did understand that nourishing the body was the way to achieve balance. Because Marilyn did not go on a low-calorie diet, she did not set herself up for a lifetime of yo-yo dieting, like Elizabeth. More important, Marilyn did not cut fat but went on a balanced eating program that was sufficient in proteins and fats.

Childhood body-fat gain and fatigue are early markers in the accelerated metabolic aging process. Balanced nutrition and sufficient exercise are the ways to reverse this process—not calorie-restrictive or low-fat dieting! Balancing your child's nutrition and exercise is something you must do together as a family. Eating meals together and having the right snacks available is important. In my experience, children prefer real food when they get rid of the "noise" in their heads that demands junk and processed products.

Vegetarianism is a growing trend in American children. I do not discourage people from eating a vegetarian diet. But the vegetarian diet can have serious consequences if not followed properly. Morris's story, in chapter 21, illustrates how damaging a poor vegetarian diet can be.

PART VI

The Vegetarian Diet

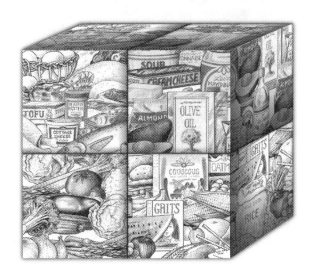

Twenty-One

The Committed Vegetarian

M orris, a fifty-five-year-old man, came to me specifically for a follow-up visit and checkup of his pituitary hormones. As usual when anyone comes to see me, we discussed eating habits. Morris ate a vegetarian diet. Like many of my vegetarian patients, he was eating an excess of carbohydrates and not enough proteins and fats.

Morris: I had a pituitary tumor removed five years ago, and then my endocrinologist moved and I needed to find another doctor. That was my primary reason for going to see Dr. Schwarzbein.

I've been a vegetarian for sixteen years. During those years I didn't eat any dairy products at all. Nor did I eat eggs for several years. Then I realized that by eating baked goods I was getting some eggs. So I started eating eggs again, but I would have just the whites. Sometimes if I ate out I'd have an omelet—with dry toast, of course. I intentionally avoided fat all those years. I never had butter in the house.

My cholesterol was slowly rising. It started to become noticeable, even alarming. In the last five years or so my total cholesterol was 225, then 250, and it went up all the way to 283. I was doing all the "right things," and it kept going up. I thought I had a pretty good diet, based upon what everybody else was talking about. In spite of the way I was eating, I had gained fat around my middle and my cholesterol was climbing. I couldn't understand it.

My wife, Stephanie, was seeing Dr. Schwarzbein for menopause issues and was talking about her approach to nutrition. Stephanie does not eat a vegetarian diet.

I was appalled when I first heard about the diet. It just didn't make any sense to me. When Stephanie told me she was going to have eggs every day, I couldn't believe it. I said, "This is contrary to what everybody else is saying." Of course it was totally opposite from the way I was eating. I was not eating any meat. I was getting protein from eating tofu occasionally, but not every day. I was eating lots of carbs. I mean lots.

My typical breakfast was oatmeal, toast and a banana. All carbs. Instead of using milk in my cereal, I used apple juice. I knew sugar wasn't good, but I thought food was not sugar. Honey's not sugar. Rice and bread are certainly not sugar. Only refined sugar is sugar, right? Dinner and lunch were steamed vegetables and rice. Lots of fruit and fresh vegetables. I was eating a high-carb, low-fat diet.

I understood that it was good to eat all the fruit you could. If I was hungry I would eat more fruit. And then I craved more. Sometimes I would go the whole day, skip lunch and eat only fruit. I figured that's good, it's healthy. How could I go wrong? But I was gaining fat.

I'm a sporadic exerciser. I love to work. I'm one of those guys who sits down at his desk, you know, screwed to the chair.

I've never had a protein deficiency, or so I thought. I was told that your body gets enough protein in non-animal foods. I understood that Dr. Schwarzbein was big on proteins and fats, and I was very resistant to that. But since Stephanie was raving about her program, I decided to give it a shot. By the time I went to see Dr. Schwarzbein in September of 1995, I was more open to hearing about the program.

Dr. Schwarzbein: Morris could not understand why he was gaining fat around his middle or why his cholesterol levels were abnormal. I explained to him that all carbohydrates are perceived as sugar in the body.

His breakfast was nothing more than one big sugar meal. Skipping meals and eating fruit caused his insulin levels to rise, putting him on the accelerated metabolic aging track, which resulted in fat around his middle and high cholesterol numbers.

People go on a vegetarian diet to avoid eating animal products. But many people do not focus on how to eat a balanced diet that includes sufficient protein. Most vegetarians today eat cereal with soy milk for breakfast, or pancakes, fruit and orange juice. Lunch is usually a salad, and dinner consists of pasta or rice with beans. In between, they snack on sweets, low-fat cookies, low-fat pretzels, rice cakes and so on. People believe that they are eating well if they do not eat animal products or if they do not gain "weight."

However, many people do not stay trim on a vegetarian diet. There are a lot of vegetarians, like Morris, who gain body fat and wonder what they can possibly be doing wrong. The answer is simple: They are eating too many carbohydrates, and this excess sugar raises insulin levels. As you know by now, insulin is the fat-storing hormone. On a high-carbohydrate diet, your body composition will gradually become more fat with less lean body mass.

People who hear about my program of higher protein instantly assume that everyone has to eat animal products to do the program correctly. Not so. You can eat a vegetarian diet. The key is to do it right. Getting the proper amount of protein and fats is essential. This takes effort because a vegetarian diet does not offer as many protein choices, and our society is geared to fast and accessible carbohydrates.

Morris: I started eating one or two eggs every morning for breakfast, with less carbs. I started eating a little cheese. I didn't go overboard. I didn't go on a high-fat diet, but I included more fat in my diet, whereas before I was eating almost none. I cut back on my fruit intake because I had been eating it recreationally. I reduced my number of carbs per meal. I ate that way for three months. The first thing I noticed was that my sugar cravings went down immediately.

Dr. Schwarzbein: Like Morris, you can eat a vegetarian diet and meet your body's need for protein and fats. But it takes some effort. If you do not eat eggs, then eating tofu is a good way to get your daily protein. The firm type of tofu has twice the protein per serving size as the softer variety. However, unlike eggs, tofu is not a complete protein. A complete protein is one that contains enough of all of the ten essential amino acids. Tofu does not contain enough of the essential amino acid methionine. You can get methionine from amaranth, barley, corn, buckwheat and brazil nuts. If you are eating tofu instead of eggs, it is important to combine foods correctly to obtain enough of all the essential amino acids.

People often tell me that they are getting a complete protein when they eat rice and beans together. It is true that rice and beans together make a complete protein. However, look at the protein-to-carbohydrate ratio in rice and beans:

One cup of brown rice = 5 grams of protein/
46 grams of carbohydrate

One cup of kidney beans = 15 grams of protein/
40 grams of carbohydrate

Total: *20 grams of protein/*
86 grams of carbohydrate

This food combination causes insulin levels to rise too high. Still, it is better to eat legumes and grains together than to eat pasta and salad, because pasta is not a protein but is a man-made carbohydrate and causes insulin levels to rise even higher.

Morris: The results were astounding. Eating eggs every day, my cholesterol dropped a hundred points. I said, "What the heck is this?" I didn't lose that much weight, maybe six to ten pounds, but I lost several inches.

Dr. Schwarzbein: As with the other case histories you have read in previous chapters, Morris lost fat and gained more muscle mass on the diet program I prescribed. This is the reason he lost inches instead of weight. Muscle weighs more than fat.

Morris: I kind of fell off the wagon after awhile when everything got really good. You know, I said, "Oh well, everything's great now so I can lighten up a little bit." So I had dessert every now and then and some wine. The sugar's the killer. There's no question about it. It's not the fat; it's the sugar. When I started to indulge, I started to gain fat again.

When I have dessert or another glass of wine, then all of a sudden the cravings are there again. I like coffee. If I have an occasional cup of coffee, that occasional cup becomes one cup a day. I find that I want more. So I have more. Then I have to stop altogether. It's the same thing with sweets. If I am going to have a sweet, I'm going to have a nice pastry or some good ice cream. I try to keep sugar to zero, but you can't go overboard. I say, "Okay, I'm going to break the rules every now and then, but it's not going to become every day."

Dr. Schwarzbein: Since the body's systems are interconnected, not only can proper nutrition correct many disorders, it can literally save your life. Unfortunately, for various reasons, some people cannot follow the program as faithfully as they should. Morris, for example, enjoys drinking coffee and eating desserts occasionally.

Everyone reacts differently to changing eating habits. I advise my patients to do the best they can and to not feel guilty if they are not perfect. Any improvements you make in your eating and lifestyle habits will make a difference. Try to define why you are having such a tough time. If you crave carbohydrates and succumb to eating comfort foods, then you must address your low-serotonin state by supplying your body with adequate proteins and fats to make serotonin and by taking the supplements recommended in chapter 4.

If you have gone on the healing program by increasing proteins and fats and decreasing carbohydrates, make sure you are eating enough carbohydrates. Carbohydrate craving can be caused by reducing carbohydrate consumption too much, which deprives your body of energy and leads to low serotonin levels. Conversely, eating *too many* carbohydrates sets up hypoglycemic cycles. (See chapter 18 for more on hypoglycemia.) If drinking coffee and eating pastry are a habitual problem, keep working on including more fats and proteins in your diet and avoiding man-made carbohydrates. The sooner you feed your body what it really needs and wants, the sooner your carbohydrate cravings will disappear. If you need to eat something sweet, choose fruit—or at least real food products like real ice cream, for example. Stay away from chemically processed and low-fat desserts.

If your carbohydrate cravings do not go away or become worse on this program, you may have a hormonal imbalance that needs to be addressed.

If you want to eat a vegetarian diet, you must make sure you are combining foods that will give you complete proteins and you must eat enough of them. You must also address your body's need for essential fats by eating good oils. It is very tough to eat a healthy vegetarian diet in today's world, especially here in the United States, where we have gotten so far away from real, wholesome foods.

Again, I never discourage anyone from eating a vegetarian diet. I discourage eating a bad vegetarian diet of cereals, pasta, breads and sweets. *A good vegetarian diet emphasizes tofu, seeds, legumes, nuts and whole grains, such as barley and quinoa, to get all the protein you need. A good vegetarian diet also provides essential fats from avocados, olives and oils.* You must mix and balance foods to get the needed nutritional balance at every meal. It is more work to eat a good vegetarian diet than it is to eat a meat-based diet, but it can be done.

People have different reasons for committing to the vegetarian diet. In chapter 22, you will read about Sarah, who followed a vegetarian diet only because she believed that meat products were unhealthy.

Twenty-Two

The Body Is Interconnected

Sarah is a soft-spoken, intelligent forty-four-year-old woman who came to see me about her weight and health issues. She was on a vegetarian diet and was struggling with excessive body fat. Having read a local newspaper article about my views on nutrition, she began by telling me that what she had read made sense and she wanted to hear more.

Sarah: I was a real skinny kid until I was five. Then all of a sudden, I was a chubby little kid. It didn't help that my mother had beautiful twin daughters when I was six. My father always held it against me that I was fat. His daughters' purpose was to be gorgeous and to glorify him to his friends.

My mother put me on diet pills when I was nine. They were amphetamines. I couldn't sleep at night. I'd go downstairs and watch the Jack Parr show while my mother ironed. My dad would say, "She's just trying to get attention." After a month, my mother finally said, "Well, if she just wants attention, she wouldn't be keeping it up this long." I went off those pills. My next diet was with food exchanges. The family would get dinner and I'd get a little muffin pan with little portions in it. I rebelled. I said, "I'm not going to do this."

I started my period at twelve. I didn't have regular periods and never did. I would skip as many as three months at a time. I also had bad menstrual cramps. Also when I was twelve, they tested me for an underactive thyroid and put me on thyroid supplements all through high school. But it didn't help my weight.

Weight Watchers was my idea. I was in my senior year and weighed 220 pounds. The old Weight Watchers back in the late sixties was heavy on protein—an entire can of tuna fish or four hot dogs at a time and restricted carbs. I got down to about 170 before I went to college.

I got married after college and gained a lot of weight. I started eating a macrobiotic diet then. I didn't lose, but I didn't gain. I believed that the macrobiotic diet was helpful because it got me over obvious sugar foods, but ultimately it was really unhelpful because it focused a lot on other carbohydrates.

At thirty-three, I went back to school, started working and got divorced. I met my second husband-to-be when I was thirty-five. As my life stabilized and I got happier, I started eating again and gained weight. I tried Weight Watchers again but this time it didn't work for me. Looking back, the program was different so that you got a lot more carbs and not as much protein as their original program.

Because my fiancé had high cholesterol, we then switched to a low-fat diet—skim milk, low-fat cottage cheese. We both gained more weight right away.

I lost my parents, both my grandmothers and my stepmother, all within a four-year period. I gained more weight. My fiancé and I moved to Santa Barbara. I gained even more weight.

My weight has been a constant struggle. I'm five feet, nine inches tall. In my adult life, my weight has ranged from 160 to 320 pounds. I never really got a measure of peace until I read a feminist book on being fat. I started to question why I should be held to different standards than men. I have had my share of pain from being denied jobs and having people hang out of cars and scream insults at me. People say really hurtful things. Fat is one of the last easy targets for people to discriminate against. It's still okay in our society to believe that it's disgusting to be fat and to outright discriminate against people on the basis of that.

You have to listen to yourself when it comes to healing. I really couldn't figure out what to eat, so I turned vegetarian. But everything I ate seemed to give me cravings. I was never satisfied. I'd eat some of this; no, that didn't feel right. Eat some of that; no, that didn't feel right either. I bounced all over. I thought, *I just have to find some solution where I'm not thinking about food all the time. This is no way to live.*

I read an article about Diana Schwarzbein in the newspaper. There were follow-up letters to the editors and people saying, "Oh, this one's a quack," and, "You're all going to die of heart disease eating that much fat." But there was something that made sense to me about what she said in the interview. It occurred to me that when I was a chubby kid, everybody said, "Just cut back on her starches." You know, don't eat the potatoes, don't eat the bread. Something kicked in, too, about this low-fat stuff. I knew it didn't work for me. Also, I remember my mother always insisting that you should eat butter, not margarine. You know, that's how it came out of the cow, and the cow knows best. This sense of whole food—not tampering with food—appealed to me.

I thought, too, that if I wanted to eat vegetarian then I had better go and find out how to do that right. Besides wanting help with my diet, I was feeling really old. I was at my highest weight, 320. I was having lots of physical problems—pains in my joints, muscle pain, fatigue, headaches.

I went to see Dr. Schwarzbein a year and five months ago. She explained about insulin and metabolism. It made sense. I have a degree in biology, so I understood what she was saying. So when she talked about insulin resistance, it registered, because in my family there was Type II diabetes, and I was very fatigued when I ate sugar.

Dr. Schwarzbein: Ultimately, Sarah decided that she didn't want to stay with the vegetarian diet. She had stopped eating meat and poultry only because she thought they were unhealthy.

I asked her to go on the healing program. Because she was very anxious about her weight and wanted to see quick results, I was somewhat concerned that she would go too low in her carbohydrate consumption. I explained that a zero-gram carbohydrate diet would cause a rapid lowering of insulin levels, which would likely lead to decreased production of serotonin, causing fatigue, depression, insomnia, increased appetite and headaches.

Sarah: I started eating meat again right away. I got out all my old cook-books—all the recipes I hadn't been cooking because they either had too much fat in them or meat. Steamed asparagus with cream cheese wrapped in prosciutto. Hamburgers, for gosh sakes—without the buns of course, but it was really neat. It was fun to eat again and not feel bad about it. I kept food diaries, and when Dr. Schwarzbein looked them over she'd say, "Well, I think you need to eat more." It was the first time in my life a doctor told me to eat more. It was wonderful news.

In addition to the eating program, Dr. Schwarzbein had me start walking. In fact, exercise has become as important as what I'm eating. I'm walking, biking and doing tai chi almost daily. I've lost fat and feel a lot more energetic. The fat loss was great, but I gained muscle, too. People are starting to notice and remark that I'm getting smaller. My legs and stomach are smaller. I'm starting to get a lap now!

My triglycerides, cholesterol and blood pressure all have significantly improved. This is the first time in my life that I've had monthly periods. I became regular within two months of starting on this program, and it's been that way ever since. I now understand that the whole body works together.

Dr. Schwarzbein: In medical school there were two schools of thought: There were the "separators" and the "lumpers." Separators saw each system and mechanism of the human body as separate entities. Of course I was a lumper, because it was clear to me that all systems and mechanisms of the human body were interconnected, not only by bones and tissues but by hormones and other chemical communicators. As a lumper, I believe that you need to do only a few simple things to stay healthy. One important thing is to keep insulin levels balanced.

The human body is complex, and obviously problems can arise from factors other than insulin imbalances, but think of insulin as the front domino piece. If that domino piece topples over, it starts a cascade of problems. Keeping that domino piece steady is the key to good health.

Of course there is a lot more science about the human body than can be explained in one book. The most important thing for you to remember from reading this book is that everything you put into your mouth is going to affect insulin in some way. When insulin levels are kept high too long, you end up with a physiology that promotes blood clots, heartburn, irritable bowel, allergies, asthma and inflammation, osteoarthritis, different types of cancer, cholesterol abnormalities, coronary artery disease, less lean body mass with excess body fat, high blood pressure, osteoporosis, stroke, Type II diabetes, and earlier death. When insulin levels are kept too low (by overexercising and not eating enough food), you will waste away and suffer from low serotonin (depression, fatigue, insomnia and so on) and osteoporosis.

Sarah: I'm not sure how much weight I've lost—though I've gone down four sizes. I don't own a scale. Weight isn't the issue now. I'm much more at peace with myself. For the first time in my life I really don't resent my body. I had always felt like I was at war with my body. To lose weight and keep it off took so much mental effort. Who wants to make food the center of your life? If I never lost another pound, I'd be happy. Going through life in a constant struggle of will to deny yourself something that you want is no way to live. So it's a liberation. Food is more of a fun, nurturing thing now. The healing program restored my trust in my body and taught me balance.

The experiences of Benjamin, Robert, Vanessa, Joel, Miriam, Riley, Gordon, Charles, Elizabeth, myself, Vickie, Alex, Marilyn, Morris and Sarah all demonstrate that human beings are meant to be part of nature. When you step away from nature and eat man-made products, ingest chemicals and deprive your body of proteins and fats, two of the most essential nutrient groups, you enter an accelerated aging process that leads to chronic degenerative diseases. Because illness and aging are outcomes of the same process, anyone's metabolism can be ruined by a diet and lifestyle that cause the person to become ill.

Like everyone else, Sarah, too, significantly improved her health through the healing program. Her lifestyle took a dramatic turn for the better. As Sarah continues on the healing program, she will achieve optimum health and reach her ideal body composition.

Even though you may want to take responsibility and do the right thing for your health, the idea of changing your lifestyle may seem impossible. Chapter 23 in part VII tells the story of Beth, who changed her lifestyle painlessly.

PART VII

Changing Your Lifestyle

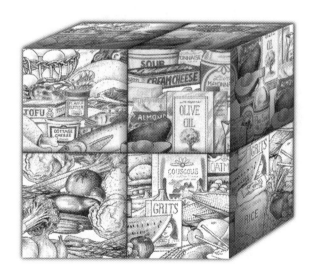

Twenty-Three

Changing Her Lifestyle
Without Suffering

B y now you have probably come to the conclusion that you have some work to do on your lifestyle. Maybe you have tried to change your lifestyle with other programs and found that sooner or later your motivation fizzled out. You did not see results fast enough, or it was too hard to sustain, or there was simply not enough return for all the effort you put in. Beth, a forty-two-year-old registered nurse, believed that it was impossible to change her lifestyle. No matter how much she wanted to change or how much she tried, she always fell back into her old ways.

Beth: When I was young, I had this illusion that if I was thinner or got my act together, my life would improve somehow and I would be happier. I finally got wise enough to realize that it wasn't just one thing, like losing weight, that would make me happy.

I had pretty much given up the notion that there would ever be a way for me to change my lifestyle. I've done every diet. Every program. Nothing ever worked. I have friends who have healthy regimens, but it seems to me they've always lived healthy lifestyles for as long as I've known them. It isn't like they changed their habits at any point. On the other hand, when I tried to find examples of people going from one way of being and eating and living to another, I couldn't find any. I had tried so many different things. I'm intelligent and have the ability to commit to things. I work very hard. But I've never been able to open the door that would enable me to change my lifestyle. So I thought the idea of changing your lifestyle was a joke. It's impossible and most people can't do it.

I heard about Dr. Schwarzbein and her healing program, and I thought I would go see what she had to say. I am six feet tall and weighed 335 when I went to see her.

I'm a nurse, and I happen to like physiology a lot. When Dr. Schwarzbein explained what she knew about nutrition, I got very excited because it made sense to me. A lot of what she said about other ways of dieting and weight loss I had empirically discovered for myself—basically nothing worked to assure any permanent weight loss.

So I got some hope just from her explanation of the program and why it worked. Dr. Schwarzbein asked me why I wanted to do the program. I said I didn't think that following the program would make my life better. I wasn't going to be any happier if I lost weight; I am pretty happy with my life as it is. I have a husband and great kids and a career, and I didn't need to be thinner for that. So I said, "I'd like to fit in an airline seat. I fly all the time and I would like to be comfortable sitting next to people on the airplane." It's something people don't talk about—the discomfort of being larger than the size that everything is built for.

I started on the program. My husband and I had eggs every morning— omelets with turkey, ham, onions, mushrooms, tomato and cheese, cooked in butter. Low-carb toast with butter. I do nutritional analysis in my work. So I have a computer program where you can put in what a person eats and it spits out the results. I put in the numbers for our breakfast one morning. In terms of cholesterol and fats, it was five times the daily recommended requirements.

I called Dr. Schwarzbein and I asked, "Are you sure this is okay?"

She said, "Yes, this is exactly what I want you to do."

I continued on the program and felt something really different within the first month. I'm not even talking about weight loss. I mean emotionally. I went in and talked to Dr. Schwarzbein and said, "What is going on? I feel like I'm on some kind of happy drug."

Dr. Schwarzbein: I explained to Beth that with proper nutrition comes balance. Part of the balance is a sense of well-being. Until Beth started the healing program, her diet was deficient in proteins and fats. On a protein-deficient diet, her brain never produced a steady supply of serotonin. When she ate properly, her body began to improve serotonin production and her mood improved. Also, eating balanced meals balanced out every hormone system in her body. *Because the body is interconnected, one balance leads to another balance.*

Beth: I've never been a binge eater. I've never had any eating disorder like bulimia or anorexia or that kind of thing. But I would have these hour-and-a-half to two-hour cycles of starving a very short time after I ate. Then I would try to satisfy the hunger or, if I was on a diet, try not to satisfy it. I had never felt what it was like to eat and be satisfied. On this program, I felt a sense of peace from not being controlled by food and hunger. It was great to be free of the struggle of trying not to eat when I was hungry.

I found it really very easy to follow this program. I don't even like to call it a diet or a program because it's not. I am not perfect at it either. I just watch the carbohydrates. I pay really close attention to that. One of the first things I remember is this feeling of evenness—of being satisfied or satiated. I don't go to the refrigerator and open the door and stare anymore, trying to figure out what I want.

In the past I never had the energy to do anything that would be considered a lifestyle change. Slowly I'm doing physical stuff. That's a big change for me, because I've never been able to maintain any physical activity beyond little spurts of effort. I never had the energy for it.

I've played racquetball for years—you can actually play racquetball standing pretty still. You either get the ball or you don't, but you don't have to put a lot of effort into it. And so I started that up again. I started walking, too. Then I thought, well, the goal here is to build muscle, so lifting weights would probably be a really good thing to do. I started to have the energy for that, too, so I started lifting weights.

The old diet mentality is to have this fear that if you go off your diet, you're going to fall by the wayside. Because you usually do. But I don't have cravings and I don't miss anything. I like popcorn at the movies. So I take my string cheese to eat first, and I go ahead and have popcorn at the movies. It's a lot more carbs than I'm supposed to be having for a snack, but I have it when I feel like it. I'm not afraid that I'm ever going to stop the program. I will lose more body fat because I'm going to keep eating like this.

I lost forty-five pounds in the first five months. When I saw Dr. Schwarzbein a couple of weeks ago I said, "Miraculously, all the airlines have made their seats bigger. And the movie theaters, too, and the restaurants."

My true weight loss is not reflected by what the scale is showing, though I've lost a total of seventy pounds. Besides losing body fat, I have built up all this muscle. I am much trimmer than I was at this same weight before. My clothes size is also smaller than it was when I weighed this amount. In fact, I'm just about to get rid of about half my wardrobe because I have dropped more than four sizes. But weight loss is not the most important thing.

It's so easy for people to say, "Oh, another way to lose weight. Or another way to get happy." But what I want to emphasize is that I feel like a normal person for the first time in my life. I've always been driven and hyper, and I always kind of associated that with my personality. Well, I can see now it wasn't just my personality. I was on this yo-yo of emotions, being driven all the time by this uneven life of never feeling right. I can't ever imagine doing anything different from this for the rest of my life. It hit me that I actually had changed my lifestyle, which I really didn't think was possible. It's been pretty invisible.

Dr. Schwarzbein: Beth was able to change her lifestyle without even noticing the effort. Beth's experience on the healing program summarizes what my other patients have experienced, and I could not have said it better.

You may believe that, even if you could change your eating and lifestyle habits, it is too late to make any real difference. But the truth is it is never too late. Part VIII explains how you can get started.

PART VIII

The Healing and Maintenance Programs

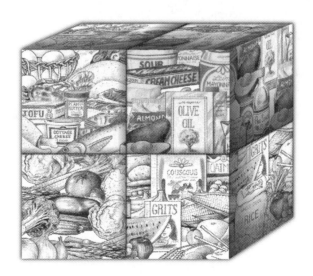

Twenty-Four

The Schwarzbein Nutrition and Lifestyle Programs

y clinical experience with over three thousand patients has demonstrated that degenerative diseases of aging are not genetic but acquired by poor eating and lifestyle habits. Since the systems of the human body are interconnected, what you do to imbalance one system creates another imbalance, which leads to accelerated aging and earlier death. My work has also shown that these imbalances can be corrected at any point in your life and that it is never too late.

As you have learned throughout this book, all hormones are linked and one hormone imbalance creates another hormone imbalance. Because this is true, we focus on achieving insulin balance as a way to achieve total hormone balance.

Any changes you make, no matter how small, will make a difference in your health. You are in control of your metabolism minute to minute, day to day, year to year. Metabolism is resilient and you can constantly redirect its course. The first course of action is to establish whether or not you are on the accelerated metabolic aging track. Check any of the following that apply to you.

Are You on the Accelerated
Metabolic Aging Track?

❑ Are you over forty years old?

❑ Have you skipped meals, dieted or yo-yo dieted (fasting, low-fat, high-carbohydrate or low-calorie)?

❑ Have you used over-the-counter drugs?

❑ Have you taken prescription drugs?

❑ Have you eaten damaged fats? (Damaged fats are trans-fatty acids, oxidized and hydrogenated fats. See detailed explanation in chapter 26.)

❑ Do you have triglyceride levels higher than 150?

❑ Are you overweight, with excess fat around the midsection ("insulin meter")?

❑ Are you underweight, with decreased muscle mass?

❑ Do you have any reactive hypoglycemic symptoms: nausea, shakiness, clamminess, sweating, lightheadedness, irritability, heart racing or anxiety?

❑ Do you have elevated blood pressure?

❑ Do you suffer from fatigue?

❑ Do you carbohydrate-crave and/or stimulant-crave?

❑ Do you suffer from insomnia/sleep disorders (such as abrupt waking)?

❑ Do you suffer from depression/mood swings/anxiety/obsessing?

❑ Do you suffer from premenstrual syndrome (PMS)?

❑ Are you perimenopausal or menopausal?

❑ Do you suffer from acne, allergies, asthma, chronic pain, chronic yeast infections, headaches, infertility, intestinal disturbances, joint aches and/or pains?

❑ Do you suffer from a low libido?

❑ Do you have any of the degenerative diseases of aging: osteoarthritis, any type of cancer, cholesterol abnormalities, coronary artery disease, less lean body mass with excess body fat, high blood pressure, osteoporosis, stroke or Type II diabetes?

Checking off several signs and symptoms means you are insulin resistant, have a lowered metabolism and are probably serotonin depleted. As you learned in chapter 1, the key to longevity is delaying insulin resistance for as long as possible. If you are already insulin resistant, however, you can begin reversing this process by eliminating eating and lifestyle habits that increase insulin levels.

Checking off the degenerative diseases indicates that your metabolism is extremely damaged. But there is hope, because, as I explained above, it is never too late to regain your health. However, if you already have a degenerative disease, you cannot afford to wait another day. You must begin the regeneration process immediately.

Do you have high-insulin habits? Check the following that apply to you.

Habits That Raise Insulin Levels

❑ Do you eat a low-fat diet?

❑ Do you yo-yo diet?

❑ Do you skip meals?

❑ Do you eat excess carbohydrates (including man-made and refined sugar)?

❑ Do you use saccharin, aspartame (artificial sweeteners), margarine or any other invented substances, refined and processed foods?

❑ Do you eat damaged fats? (Damaged fats are trans-fatty acids, oxidized and hydrogenated fats. See detailed explanation in chapter 26).

❑ Do you use caffeine (coffee, tea, sodas, chocolate)?

❑ Do you drink soft drinks?

❑ Do you drink alcohol?

❑ Do you use tobacco?

❑ Do you use natural stimulants such as ma huang?

❑ Do you use recreational stimulants (amphetamines, cocaine, heroin)?

❑ Are you stressed?

❑ Are you sedentary?

❏ Do you take prescription drugs?

❏ Do you take excessive and/or unnecessary thyroid hormone medication or Armour thyroid?

❏ Do you take steroids?

❏ Do you take over-the-counter cold medications?

❏ Do you use diet pills?

❏ Do you take dextroamphetamine sulfate (Dexedrine) or methylphenidate hydrochloride (Ritalin)?

Balanced insulin levels are essential to reversing insulin resistance, improving metabolism and correcting a low-serotonin state. The following habits will lower high insulin levels to normal.

Habits That Lower Insulin Levels

The following will lower your insulin levels:

Reversing the above bad habits

Exercise

Eating good oils and fats

Eating good fiber (vegetables)

Taking hormone replacement therapy, if needed

The purpose of reversing bad habits is to get your insulin levels from high to normal. This may seem impossible if you have many bad habits. Sometimes people cannot change everything at once. You should work on what you can. Do your best and remember that everything you do to improve your eating and lifestyle habits will bring you closer to optimum health. Here are a few words of encouragement:

Do not feel guilty or stressed-out over your current habits.

You do not need to change all your habits at once.

Begin slowly, one step at a time.

Give yourself credit for every positive change you are able to make.

The Schwarzbein Nutrition and Lifestyle Program addresses five issues that are intrinsically linked to good health:

Nutrition

Stress Management

Exercise

Eliminating Stimulants and Other Drugs

Hormone Replacement Therapy

Step I: Nutrition

People correlate being healthy with being thin. By now you know that being thin is not synonymous with good health. Our society has developed destructive methods in trying to achieve health through weight loss. Low-fat dieting, starvation dieting, liquid diets, fasting, skipping meals, counting calories, diet pills (including prescription) and so on have put people on the metabolic aging track and have caused the rise in disease over the past twenty years.

The Goal: Optimum Health

The purpose of the Schwarzbein Program is to get you off the metabolic aging track and to reeducate you about good health. It is important for you to understand that "weight loss" is not the goal. *The goal is optimum health.* One of the many benefits you will enjoy along with optimum health is an ideal body composition.

The body type you will achieve with balanced nutrition and lifestyle may not be the body type you have learned to accept as "ideal." Because our culture has adopted an unhealthy ideal of women looking like prepubescent girls, we are led to believe that any amount of flesh lying over our bones is too much. I have women patients who are chronic dieters, who are thin and think they look good. But their bodies are not sleek and well-toned. Instead, with the loss of lean body mass, they have slack skin over lumpy fat deposits (or worse, over hollow bones). This body type is achieved through deprivation and torturous workouts. Although it is not attractive or healthy, many women are so fixated on the number on the scale and on calorie and fat-gram counting that they do not recognize how their bodies actually look. As long as they fit into their size-three to size-five clothes, they are happy.

Likewise, men have gotten into trouble trying to prevent heart disease. Men typically are not as body conscious as women, but they are worried about dying prematurely from a heart attack. They have bought into believing that all they need to do is eliminate cholesterol and fat from their diet and they will live longer. But deprivation and workouts have not given us ideal bodies or prevented heart attacks. Instead, they have caused us to be on the accelerated metabolic aging track.

One of the Benefits: Ideal Body Composition

The true ideal body composition that humans should strive for is one of sleek, toned muscle and solid bones. This body composition is not attainable through starvation and extreme exercise. In fact, you *must eat* to become healthy and to lose body fat. You cannot lose body fat by fasting or going hungry without damaging your metabolism. The Schwarzbein Program will put you back on the path to optimum health and ideal body composition through a combination of balanced nutrition, exercise, eliminating stimulants and other drugs, stress management, and hormone replacement therapy, if needed.

You have tried the alternatives (restricting calories or fat) and know what those results are. If you want good health and an ideal body composition, you must give this program time. During the healing process you will notice dramatic improvements in the way you feel: improved sleep, more energy and vitality, better concentration and memory, improved moods, improved immune function, less carbohydrate craving and improved libido. These are all important signals that you are on your way to optimum health.

On the healing program, most excessively overweight people will lose weight at the rate of one to two pounds a week. This is because not all overweight people have completely destroyed their metabolism. Even though they might have an excessive amount of fat, they also have muscle underneath. The more muscle mass you have, the more capable your metabolism is of burning fat.

Other overweight people will not see a change in their weight for six months to a year. As they heal their metabolism, they build muscle mass that eventually begins to burn off fat stores. Even though you may not notice changes in your weight, your body will begin to look and feel different.

If you are very thin or have destroyed your metabolism by various weight-loss efforts, you will initially gain pounds (muscle, bone and fat) on this program. Of course, you may find any weight gain alarming. But remember, there is going to be a lag time between where you are now metabolically and where you want to be. It took years to destroy your metabolism, and you will have to go through a healing period to restore your health. As your insulin resistance is corrected (by building lean body mass and by emptying cells of excess sugar), *and* as you continue to eat enough food so that your body understands the time of famine is over, you will begin to lose body fat and reach your ideal body composition. (See "Millions of Years of Genetics Can Work Against You," page 152.)

If you become discouraged at any point along the way, remember that there is no other method of achieving health and an ideal body composition except through balanced nutrition and lifestyle changes.

My staff and I have encouraged many men and women through the initial healing stages of this program. The good news is that everyone who stays with the program is ultimately very happy with the results.

If you begin the healing program after many years of dieting, you may not be able to eat the amount of food prescribed without suffering from indigestion, bloating, gas, constipation and water retention. Using digestive enzymes such as papaya tablets, and taking a stress-fighting B-complex with breakfast and 500 milligrams of magnesium at bedtime, will help you through this adjustment period.

Men will usually achieve faster results in their health and body composition than women, because men have more lean body mass to begin with and fewer hormone imbalances.

> It is important to emphasize that optimum health is not achieved by losing "weight." Shifting your focus from the number on the scale to the real factors of good health, such as improved mood, energy and vitality, is the way to accomplish a lifetime of balance *and* your ideal body composition.

All of the good effects of the healing program may not happen immediately. If you are following this program and you do not feel better or see any improvements in your health, you might not be eating correctly. In such a case, a food diary can be helpful. My patients often tell me that they are appalled at their diets when they honestly write down everything they eat. For this reason, a journal can help you isolate and improve your problem areas while allowing you to decide if you need more fat, protein, vegetables or even more carbohydrates in your diet. It will also help you determine your needs in the areas of exercise, eliminating stimulants and other drugs, managing your stress and taking hormone replacement therapy.

Step II: Stress Management

Stress is harmful because stress imbalances every hormone system of your body. The imbalances from stress are apparent in the terrible way you feel during periods of stress or right after a stressful situation. To achieve optimum health and an ideal body composition, you must focus on regular stress management to keep insulin and other hormone levels balanced.

Everyday stress can feel overwhelming. But there are many ways to find relief in our stressful world. When you focus on stress management, you will find that you feel a greater sense of balance.

In addition to everyday stress, events occur that are outside of your control: the death of a loved one, losing your job, going through a divorce, for example. Sometimes you cannot manage the stress that comes along with these events. During times of undue stress, it is important to remember to take care of your body. Try not to turn to comfort foods because you feel you do not have time to focus on balanced nutrition. Times of stress require even more diligence to keep your eating and lifestyle habits balanced. If you are faced with a stressful situation, take a few minutes to mentally review what you can do to keep yourself healthy. During a crisis, friends typically ask what they can do to help. Ask a friend to help you grocery shop and prepare meals, join you for a daily walk or to be there when you need company.

Stress is a fact of life. However, it is up to you to do what you can to manage your particular stress in the best way suited to you. If stress is a major factor in your life, you must seek out professional counseling. Below are some common-sense suggestions for lowering stress for those of you with everyday stressors. Any of the activities that appeal to you can be incorporated into your lifestyle. Serotonin supplements can help (see chapter 4 for recommended supplements).

Some Ways to Lower Stress

- Acupuncture
- Adopt a cat, dog or other pet
- Aromatherapy

- Assertiveness training classes
- Avoid stressful television programs
- Balance your work schedule with adequate relaxation time
- Biofeedback therapy
- Dancing
- Develop affection in relationships (laughing, hugging, being together)
- Eat dinner with your family on a regular basis
- Forget old grudges
- Get adequate sleep
- Go to the movies more often
- Group therapy (or men's/women's group)
- Individual counseling (psychologist or spiritual counselor)
- Have a massage
- Join a book club
- Join a health club
- Join a knitting group
- Learn to delegate
- Learn to practice yoga
- Learn to say no
- Make smart job choices and do what you can to find a career you enjoy
- Meditate
- Meet friends for breakfast, lunch or dinner
- Play sports (join a team that meets regularly)
- Pray
- Reach out to someone else in need
- Take a stress-management class
- Take a long, hot bath
- Take a ten-minute walk at break time or a morning walk in your favorite place
- Take an adult education class on a subject you have always wanted to learn

- Take rest-and-relaxation periods during the day
- Take up a new hobby
- Treat yourself (buy a book or some clothes, get your hair done, have a manicure or a facial)

Step III: Exercise

Exercise is a vital component of the Five Step Program. Exercise heals your metabolism by reversing insulin resistance.

It is important to eat the right amount of carbohydrates for your current metabolism and activity level. When you exercise, you can increase your carbohydrate intake. However, you cannot reduce your carbohydrate consumption to a dangerously low level to justify not exercising. This will lead to hormone imbalances, and, if you do lose "weight" it will be lean body mass, not fat, which leads to further metabolic aging. In other words, you cannot reverse accelerated metabolic aging by only changing your eating habits.

Even though we know the health benefits of exercise, I have heard people remark about how difficult it is to get motivated. Exercise often gets put on the bottom of our list of priorities. On the other hand, those who begin and stay with an exercise program are generally the most enthusiastic advocates and are likely to make exercise a priority. The reason is that those who begin an exercise program soon discover that exercise is one sure way to improve the overall quality of their life. In fact, I can tell immediately when I meet a patient who exercises. They are younger looking, have more vitality and have fewer health problems than people who do not exercise.

It costs little or nothing to begin an exercise program. A pair of walking shoes is usually all it takes.

If you have not been exercising regularly or are tired, start slowly. Begin with an easy activity such as walking. Always stretch first to avoid injuries. Five minutes of exercise three times a day is an adequate start. Increase time in increments of five minutes, until you are up to fifteen to twenty minutes, three times a day. Three exercise periods a day is the ideal. If you do not have the time to exercise that many times in a day, exercise for one longer period or stay active in general.

If you are undernourished, have multiple health problems, or are out of shape and over the age of fifty, consult your physician for clearance to exercise. If you have multiple health problems, consider starting with an exercise rehabilitation center. Your physician can advise you which facility in your area is best for you.

The ideal time to exercise is one to two hours after eating. Ten to twenty minutes of exercise at a time is adequate.

With aerobic workouts you should aim at getting your heart rate up to 60 to 80 percent of your maximum attainable rate. A good estimate of your maximum heart rate per minute is 220 minus your age in years.

If you exercise too much when your body is undernourished, you may do more harm than good. You will know if you should be exercising, and how much, by how it makes you feel. Check your heart rate before and after.

If the exercise you have chosen thoroughly exhausts you, then it was too much for you, and too soon. Listen to your body. If it wants to rest, rest. Physical therapists, exercise physiologists and personal trainers often push too hard, especially when people are out of shape and undernourished. This leads to fatigue, muscle and ligament damage, and discouragement. Think of it this way: You would never go out and exercise if you had the flu, a cold or other illness. Think of being undernourished or out of shape in the same terms as being ill.

Do not exercise strenuously to justify overeating carbohydrates. Even if you are extremely active or athletic, you should strive to keep your meals balanced. As you learned in chapter 14, if you eat a bowl of pasta to "carbo-load" before exercising, you can "burn" off the excess sugar as energy but you cannot burn off the excess insulin that has been secreted to match the high sugar. Once insulin levels increase to a higher than normal level, damage begins to occur in your metabolism.

Do not confuse energy with stamina. To become a high-performing athlete you must build lean body mass by eating sufficient proteins and fats. A well-conditioned body performs at its optimum. Carboloading (loading up on sugar) will not result in high performance. Many studies have concluded that athletes who eat a balanced diet outperform those who eat a high-carbohydrate diet.

Equally important is that you should not overexercise, or if you are exercising strenuously, you must take care to eat enough food, in the form of balanced meals. If a woman athlete does not eat enough food she will stop menstruating or "hit the wall." If a male athlete does not eat enough food, he will "hit the wall." In other words, both men and women will fail to achieve their maximum performance without adequate nutrition.

Do not aggressively pursue an exercise you dislike. Seek out an activity you enjoy. Dancing, yoga, hiking or walking are equally good. If you cannot find the time in your schedule for structured exercise, try parking some distance from where you work or shop, take stairs and walk whenever possible. There are other simple ways to work exercise into a busy schedule by engaging in less-strenuous activities for longer periods of time, or by doing more strenuous activities in shorter spurts. For example, you could wash and wax a car for 45 to 60 minutes; wash windows or floors for 45 to 60 minutes; garden for 30 to 45 minutes; walk 2 miles in 35 minutes (20-minute mile); shoot baskets for 30 minutes; bicycle 5 miles in 30 minutes; dance fast (social) for 30 minutes or push a stroller 1.5 miles in 30 minutes. Or, if your schedule doesn't permit a long exercise period, you could do an intense activity for a shorter time period like: swim laps for 20 minutes; play wheelchair basketball for 20 minutes; bicycle 4 miles in 15 minutes; jump rope for 15 minutes; run 1.5 miles in 15 minutes (10-minute mile); shovel snow for 15 minutes; or stair walk for 15 minutes.

Step IV: Eliminating Stimulants and Other Drugs

If you crave any form of stimulants, carbohydrates or otherwise, then you are not healthy. As you have read throughout this book, you cannot achieve good health and continue to use stimulants. Stimulants raise insulin levels, lower serotonin levels and put you on the metabolic aging track.

Stimulants Found in Food

Alcohol

Caffeine

Chocolate

Ma huang

Excessive carbohydrates (especially man-made)

Sugar

Stimulants Found in Drugs

Amphetamines

Armour thyroid

Cocaine and other "recreational" drugs

Triiodothyronine (Cytomel, the active thyroid hormone)

Dextroamphetamine sulfate (Dexedrine)

Diet pills

Over-the-counter cold medications

Methylphenidate hydrochloride (Ritalin)

Phentermine (the phen in Phen Fen)

Tobacco

Although the goal is to be stimulant-free, you must taper off stimulants gradually to avoid depression and other withdrawal symptoms that would result from a rapid drop in serotonin levels. The use of stimulants is "self-medication." Therefore, it is not advisable to abruptly discontinue the use of all stimulants. As you taper off of stimulant use, if you find yourself weepy, depressed, irritable, irrational or even suicidal, increase your stimulant intake, and continue to work on restoring your serotonin levels. (See chapter 4 to learn how to restore seratonin levels.) As you become healthier, slowly begin to decrease stimulant use again. Even though the goal is to be completely stimulant-free, it is a process that takes time.

All drugs, prescription or otherwise, damage your metabolism on a cellular level. This does not mean that you should abruptly stop taking all your medications. Some people have conditions that require taking drugs. However, if applicable, discuss with your physician any lifestyle changes that would enable you to slowly taper off prescription drugs. Be your own advocate when it comes to medications, especially multiple prescriptions. Never accept a prescription for a new drug without telling your doctor all the drugs you are currently taking, including over-the-counter medications. Always question the necessity of taking any new prescription.

Step V: Hormone Replacement Therapy

If you balance your diet, manage your stress, get adequate exercise, and eliminate stimulants and other drugs and still do not reach your optimum health and ideal body composition, you may have a hormone imbalance. This is because the loss of hormones is part of the normal aging process. Seek out a physician who is well versed in hormone replacement therapy and who uses real hormones. Real hormones such as estradiol, progesterone, testosterone, levothyroxine (thyroid hormone) are identical to the hormones found in the human body. Drugs like conjugated estrogens (Premarin), medroxyprogesperone acetate (Provera) and methyltestosterone are chemicals that are not found in the human body. Armour thyroid contains real hormones but does not contain the correct composition.

The systems of the human body are interconnected, and one imbalance creates another imbalance, which leads to accelerated aging and earlier death. All the systems of the body should be balanced, including all of your hormones.

It Takes Time to Heal

I cannot stress enough that it takes time to heal your metabolism. As you read in the personal accounts throughout this book, you cannot achieve balance overnight. Consider how many years it takes to ruin a metabolism. It takes much less time to heal—nevertheless, it *does* take time. Have patience. Because healing occurs on a cellular level, it takes place from the inside out.

For most people, the hardest part is getting through the healing process. Remember, results do not appear overnight. Your body needs time to heal and repair your metabolism. Do not be discouraged. It can take more than a year to restore your metabolism. But the wait is worth it. As you follow the Schwarzbein Program of nutrition, stress management, exercise, stimulant/drug elimination and hormone replacement therapy, if needed, you will achieve a level of health you never thought possible. You will gradually notice many benefits: improved sleep, more energy and vitality, better concentration and memory, improved moods, improved immune function, less carbohydrate craving, improved libido, loss of body fat, stronger hair and nails, softer skin and hair, healing of acne, decreased irritable bowel syndrome, improved asthma, increased fertility, less bloating, less joint pain, less irritability and less PMS. These are some indicators of a well-functioning metabolism.

And remember, it is never too late.

Often, after I explain the principles of the Schwarzbein Program, my patients say, "I want to know exactly how to follow the nutritional program!" Chapter 25 will explain the nutritional healing and maintenance program in detail so that you can get off the accelerated metabolic aging track and begin enjoying the same healthy results as the patients whose experiences you have read about in this book.

Twenty-Five

The Schwarzbein Healing and Maintenance Nutritional Programs

A s you read in the interviews, I prescribe two different nutritional programs, one for healing and one for maintenance.

The Nutritional Healing Program

The nutritional healing program eliminates all sugars, chemicals and drugs. Also, it reduces carbohydrate consumption while providing needed proteins and fats so that your body can reverse insulin resistance and repair your metabolism.

During the initial stages of the healing program, you should decrease your carbohydrate consumption to slightly below your current metabolic needs (and follow the other steps of the program). This allows the cells of your body to begin to heal by using stored sugar. As cells are emptied of sugar, they replace insulin receptor doors so that insulin can once again begin to unload sugar. This is the beginning of the reversal of insulin resistance, and you are on your way to reversing accelerated metabolic aging.

To heal your metabolism you need to reduce carbohydrate

consumption and follow these basic guidelines:

- **Do not skip meals.** Five small meals a day are better than three.
- **Eat real food that you could, in theory, pick, gather, milk, hunt or fish.** Do not eat man-made carbohydrates. Do not ingest artificial sweeteners. Do not eat processed packaged foods.
- **Choose from the four nutrient groups at each meal**. Eat all the good fats and proteins your body needs. Eat a variety of non-starchy vegetables. Eat carbohydrates according to your current metabolism and activity level.
- **Taper off stimulants**. Do not consume caffeine. Do not drink alcohol. Do not ingest stimulants.
- **Avoid drugs**. Do not take any over-the-counter medications. Ask your physician if you can stop any prescription medications. (All drugs have an adverse effect at the cellular level.)

As you build muscle and repair your metabolism, you may find that you feel hungrier. This is often a stumbling block for those who have lived their entire lives depriving themselves of food when they feel hungry. Chronic dieting can turn off hunger pangs. Feeling hungry again is a good sign of renewed health. Hunger indicates your metabolism is improving and your brain needs energy. You should eat when you are hungry, but make sure that you eat proteins, fats and non-starchy vegetables. You should also eat real (not man-made) carbohydrates in a quantity that matches your activity level, current health and metabolism. When you eat fewer carbohydrates and more good fats, your insulin levels stay lower, and your body will break down its fat stores to use for energy. When you eat a balanced diet, your insulin-to-glucagon ratios are balanced. Glucagon is a fat-mobilizing hormone. In other words, glucagon "opens up" fat cells so that fat can be burned.

Some people do not feel hungry, and many people skip breakfast for this reason. It is important to eat regular meals, even if you do not feel hungry. Eventually, your body will adjust to this new healthy schedule of eating.

The Nutritional Maintenance Program

If you are on the accelerated metabolic aging track, you must begin with the *healing program*. The length of time on the healing program is determined by your individual state of health. The healing program is *not* meant to continue for the rest of your life.

Once your symptoms are alleviated or your illness is healed, the *maintenance* program prevents the same problems from recurring or new problems from developing. Following the nutritional maintenance program will keep you in good health and will delay insulin resistance. The maintenance program is also for adults and children who are already healthy and want to stay that way. The only difference between the two programs is that on the maintenance program you do not decrease carbohydrates below metabolic needs. All the other guidelines are the same.

The following section is designed to make it easy for you to switch from a low-fat, high-carbohydrate diet to a balanced diet of protein and fats, with carbohydrate consumption appropriate to your metabolism and activity level.

The Schwarzbein Four Nutrient Groups

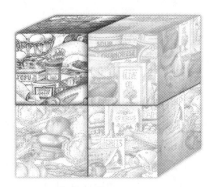

Proteins

Protein is essential for life. Eat it every day at every meal. It is not necessary to count protein grams, unless you think you are not getting enough. An ounce of animal protein contains seven grams of protein. The average minimum protein requirement for women is sixty to seventy grams per day; men need seventy to eighty grams per day.

Do not be afraid to eat more protein if your body wants it. Your body has initial feedback mechanisms to prevent you from overeating proteins and fats. (See chapter 12 for protein and fat feedback mechanisms.) Listening to your body is part of the healing process, and this will come naturally and gradually.

Select from the following choices. (Remember, you do not have to count calories or fat grams.) You should vary your selections daily.

Eggs

You can eat eggs every day, as many as your body wants.

Meat and Poultry

Whenever possible buy hormone-free, antibiotic-free, range-fed meat and poultry.

Beef	Pheasant	Quail
Chicken	Pork (bacon	Squab
Duck	and ham)[1]	Turkey
Lamb	Veal	

Additive- and Nitrate-Free Sausages

Never eat packaged sausage or lunch meats because they contain nitrates. Nitrates are used as preservatives so that supermarkets can keep meats longer than five days. Many communities have at least one old-fashioned butcher shop that still makes homemade sausage. Ask your butcher if his meats are nitrate-and additive-free. If not, request that he or she make them without nitrates.

Berliner	Chorizo	Liver sausage
Bockwurst	Duck sausage	Liverwurst
Bratwurst	Frankfurter	Polish sausage
Braunschweiger	Italian sausage	Pork sausage
(liverwurst)	Kielbasa	Pork and beef sausage
Brotwurst	Knackwurst	Turkey sausage
Chicken sausage	Liver cheese	

Paté

Chicken liver paté	Goose liver paté	Salmon paté
Duck liver paté	Rabbit liver paté	Shrimp paté

---

[1] *Bacon and ham are cured with sugar. If you must eat bacon and ham, only do so occasionally and always make sure you are buying nitrate-free meats.*

Cheese

Since most cheese is heat treated, which damages[2] the fat contained in the cheese, all cheese should be used in moderation. In addition, aged cheeses are damaged fats. Whenever possible, choose white cheese over yellow. Yellow cheeses are usually colored with artificial coloring.

The Best Cheese to Eat

Cottage cheese[3]	Goat	Neufchâtel
Cream cheese	Mozzarella (buffalo	Ricotta, whole
Feta	and regular)	or skim milk
Gjetost	Muenster	Queso fresco

Eat Only Occasionally

Bleu	Colby	Parmesan
Brick	Edam	Port de salut
Brie	Fontina	Provolone
Camembert	Gouda	Romano
Caraway	Gruyère	Roquefort
Cheddar (white only)	Limburger	Swiss
Cheshire	Monterey Jack	Tilsit

Fish and Shellfish

All fish is an excellent source of protein. Eat fresh fish instead of canned or smoked. Most smoked fish contain nitrates.

---

[2] *See chapter 26 for more on damaged fats.*
[3] *Cottage cheese, while an excellent source of protein, also contains 6 grams of carbohydrate per cup.*

Protein Foods That Contain Carbohydrates

Nuts, Nut Butters and Seeds

Nuts, nut butters and seeds are good sources of protein and fat. However, each serving below also contains six grams of carbohydrates. All items are raw unless otherwise noted. Eat nuts raw or dry roasted.

Food Item	Serving
Acorns	½ ounce
Almonds	1 ounce (23 nuts)
Almond butter	4 tablespoons
Almond paste	½ ounce
Amaranth seed	⅓ ounce
Brazil nuts (butternuts)	1½ ounces
Cashews	¾ ounce
Cashew butter	1½ tablespoons
Chinese chestnuts	½ ounce
Coconut cream	¼ cup
Coconut milk	½ cup
Coconut liquid from coconut	¾ cup
Coconut meat	½ cup, shredded
Cottonseed kernels (roasted)	1 ounce
European chestnuts	½ ounce
Filberts or hazelnuts	1½ ounces
Ginkgo nuts	½ ounce
Hickory nuts	1 ounce
Japanese chestnuts	¾ ounce
Lotus seeds	1½ ounces
Macadamia nuts	1½ ounces
Peanuts	1 ounce
Peanut butter	2 tablespoons

Food Item *(continued)*	**Serving**
Pecans	1 ounce (15 halves)
Pine nuts	1 ounce
Pistachio nuts	1 ounce (47 kernels)
Pumpkin and squash seeds	½ ounce (42 seeds)
Pumpkin and squash kernels	1 ounce (hulled)
Safflower kernels (dried)	½ ounce
Sesame butter (tahini)	1½ tablespoons
Sesame seed kernels (dried)	1 ounce
Sunflower seed kernels (dried)	¼ cup
Sunflower seed butter	1½ tablespoons
Walnuts	2 ounces
Watermelon seed kernels	⅜ cup

Soy Products

Note that while soy products are listed under protein, they also contain carbohydrates. Each of the following selections contains fifteen grams of carbohydrate.

Food Item	**Serving**
Miso (diluted)	¼ cup
Natto	½ cup
Tempeh	½ cup
Soy milk	1 cup
Soy protein	1½ ounces
Tofu[4]	1 cup

---

[4] *The firm type of tofu has more protein per ounce.*

Some Tips to Remember About Protein

• A less active lifestyle does not mean that you do not need protein. The rebuilding within your body (bones, cells, enzymes, hair, hormones, muscles, nails, neurotransmitters and so on) goes on at all times, regardless of your activity level.

• Do not eat packaged meats that contain excess salt and sugar, preservatives and nitrates. Even deli meats may contain foods prepared with additives. Ask for the ingredients before you order. Many markets are responding to the public's desire for hormone-free, antibiotic-free, range-fed meat and poultry.

• All proteins should be cooked at low, even temperatures to avoid damaged fats. (See chapter 26 for damaged fats.) Eat lean meats to avoid damaged fats.

• Buy your meat fresh, and cook and eat it within twenty-four hours. Two-day-old meat in your refrigerator has already begun to oxidize and therefore contains free radicals. (See chapter 3 for free radicals.)

Ovo-Lacto-Vegetarian Guidelines for Protein

Vegetarians must be careful to get their daily protein intake. Again, the average minimum protein requirement for a woman is sixty to seventy grams per day. The average minimum protein requirement for a man is seventy to eighty grams per day.

1 egg = 7 grams protein

1 ounce cheese = 8 to 10 grams protein

½ cup cottage cheese = 14 to 16 grams protein

1 ounce almonds = 7 grams protein

1 ounce peanuts = 7 grams protein

2 tablespoons peanut butter = 8 grams protein

½ cup tofu (firm, raw) = 20 grams protein

½ cup tempeh = 16 grams protein

Vegetarians can get their minimum daily requirement of protein by eating one cup of cottage cheese, a half cup of firm tofu, one egg and one ounce of cheese. A typical day's meals on the healing program incorporating these foods might be:

Breakfast: 1 egg, 1 slice buttered *whole-grain toast* or 2 slices buttered low-carbohydrate *toast* with 1 ounce melted cheese, topped with sliced tomato.

Lunch: Large green salad with vegetables, ½ sliced *avocado*, 1 cup cottage cheese, oil and vinegar dressing, sprinkled with *sunflower seeds* and ½ small *apple*.

Dinner: ½ cup firm tofu stir-fried with mixed vegetables, ⅓ cup buttered brown *rice*.[5]

This menu plan illustrates how easy it is for vegetarians to get their minimum daily protein requirements. However, this is not enough food for most people. I want people to eat as much food as their bodies need, while focusing on avoiding excess carbohydrates. The vegetarian meal plans on page 308 will help you plan balanced meals.

———————————

[5] *These meal plans are designed to keep your insulin-to-glucagon ratio and your glycemic index balanced (see page 122) by providing 15 grams of carbohydrate per balanced meal. While many foods contain some carbohydrate, such as tofu, they are also high in protein, fat, or fiber, and, if eaten alone, would result in a balanced insulin-to-glucagon ratio and glycemic index. It is only necessary to restrict those foods that, if they were eaten alone, would cause a rapid rise in insulin resulting in an imbalanced insulin-to-glucagon ratio and glycemic index. For that reason, only the foods that are italized are considered to contain the 15 grams of carbohydrate allowed per meal on the healing program.*

Fats

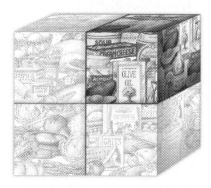

Types and Sources of Good Fats

Fats are essential for life and good health. In my experience, the more good, healthy, natural fats people eat, the healthier they become. Fats slow down the transient time of food in the digestive tract, leading to a lower glycemic index for the meal. Eat fat with every meal. Listen to your body. It knows its fat-intake limits. Do not worry about fat grams; your body takes care of this through the feedback mechanisms of satiety. If you eat too much fat, you will get sick to your stomach and possibly even vomit. You should eat as many healthy fats as you want, varying your selections.

The Difference Between Saturated, Monounsaturated and Polyunsaturated Fats

All fatty acids are made of long chains of carbon molecules hooked together. In nature, carbon must bond to four other molecules. When in a chain, carbon bonds to two other carbons, one on either side, leaving two sides unbonded.

Saturated: When these two sides are completely filled with hydrogen molecules, then the whole fatty acid is termed saturated (with hydrogen atoms).

Monounsaturated: When the whole fatty acid is missing two

hydrogen atoms, one carbon will attach twice with a carbon next to it that is also missing a hydrogen atom. This is a monounsaturated fatty acid.

Polyunsaturated: If there are other sites of hydrogens missing and other carbons attach twice to each other, then that is a polyunsaturated fatty acid.

Cross-Section of Molecules

Saturated Fatty Acid Molecule

```
    H       H       H       H       H       H       H       H
    |       |       |       |       |       |       |       |
 —  C   —   C   —   C   —   C   —   C   —   C   —   C   —   C   —
    |       |       |       |       |       |       |       |
    H       H       H       H       H       H       H       H
```

Monounsaturated Fatty Acid Molecule

```
    H       H       H       H       H       H       H       H
    |       |       |       |       |       |       |       |
 —  C   —   C   =   C   —   C   —   C   —   C   —   C   —   C   —
    |                       |       |       |       |       |
    H                       H       H       H       H       H
```

Polyunsaturated Fatty Acid Molecule

```
    H       H       H       H       H       H       H       H
    |       |       |       |       |       |       |       |
 —  C   —   C   =   C   —   C   —   C   —   C   =   C   —   C   —
    |                       |       |                       |
    H                       H       H                       H
```

Do not be afraid to eat saturated, monounsaturated or polyunsaturated fats. They are all healthy and good for you because your body is able to metabolize natural fats.

THE MYTH OF SATURATED FAT

There are many studies that vilify saturated fats. However, while conducting and analyzing the results of these studies, researchers totally ignored the fact that their subjects were eating desserts, too many carbohydrates, ingesting stimulants, not exercising enough, smoking, drinking alcohol, taking drugs and engaging in all of the other factors that cause prolonged high insulin levels. Because insulin directs all the biochemical processes that lead to plaque formation in arteries, these subjects had higher rates of heart disease.

However, my clinical experience with thousands of people has shown that eating saturated fats is not the culprit! On the contrary, the patients who I have followed, who have increased their consumption of saturated fats (as well as all other good fats), have improved their cholesterol profiles, decreased blood pressure and lost body fat, thereby reducing their risk for heart disease. Eating saturated fats should be part of your balanced diet while, at the same time, your focus should be on reducing all the factors that increase insulin levels.

Below are lists of saturated, monounsaturated and polyunsaturated fats that are good for you. Always use "pure-pressed" oils. The pure-pressing process, used to extract oil from natural sources, does not damage the fat. On the contrary, heat processes, used to extract sunflower oil from sunflower seeds, for example, damage the fat. Your body cannot metabolize any type of damaged fat. (Damaged fats are covered extensively in chapter 26.)

Saturated

Use for cooking

Butter	Cream, dairy only[6]	Nutmeg oil
Cheese	Duck fat	Sheanut oil
Chicken fat	Eggs	Sour cream
Cocoa butter	Goose fat	Turkey fat

Monounsaturated

Use for cooking

Almond oil	Grapeseed oil	Olive oil
Apricot kernel oil	Hazelnut oil	Peanut oil
Avocado oil	Mustard oil	Rice oil
Canola oil	Oat oil	

Polyunsaturated

Do not use for cooking as heat damages these fats.

Corn oil	Menhaden (fish) oil
Essential fatty acids	Salmon oil
(primrose, flaxseed,	Sardine oil
borage)	Sesame seed oil
Herring oil	Wheat germ oil

The Very Best Oils to Use

Cold or pure-pressed oil—the pure-pressing process does not create trans-fatty acids (See chapter 26 for trans-fatty acids.)

Essential fatty acids (primrose oil, flaxseed oil, borage oil)

Extra virgin olive oil is pure-pressed and therefore healthy

Fish oil

Mayonnaise made from pure-pressed canola oil and containing no hydrogenated oils

---

[6] *Some cream contains chemical additives. Only buy products labeled "dairy only."*

Some Tips to Remember About Good Fats

• A less-active lifestyle does not mean that you need less fat. The rebuilding within your body (bones, cells, enzymes, hair, hormones, muscles, nails, neurotransmitters and so on) goes on at all times, regardless of your level of activity.

• *Real* fats are life-giving substances. Do not be afraid to eat *real* fats.

• Eating fat does not make you fat, because fat does not cause the release of insulin.

• Do not use half-and-half. Use real cream, "dairy only"—not cream that contains additives.

• Saturated, monounsaturated and polyunsaturated fats are healthy. Because polyunsaturated fat is easily damaged under heat, use it at room temperature and do not cook with it.

• Do not eat any damaged fats. (See chapter 26 for damaged fats.)

Nonstarchy Vegetables

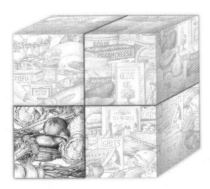

Nonstarchy vegetables provide vitamins, minerals and fiber. The vitamins and minerals in nonstarchy vegetables are used as co-enzymes, which are chemicals that speed up other chemical reactions within the body. The fibrous content of nonstarchy vegetables slows down the digestive process by taking up space in the digestive system, lowering the glycemic index of your entire meal.

It is not necessary to count the carbohydrate grams in nonstarchy vegetables because of their low glycemic index. Nonstarchy vegetables are counted as "zero" carbohydrates. Consider any vegetable portion of ½ cup that contains equal to or less than five grams of carbohydrate, to be a nonstarchy vegetable. If you are on the healing program and eat a lot of nonstarchy vegetables, you might not need to add extra carbohydrates to your meal.

Carrots are considered both a nonstarchy and a starchy vegetable. When you eat them raw, you do not have to count them as a carbohydrate because the intact fiber lowers their glycemic index. However, cooking or juicing carrots removes or breaks down the fiber, so cooked or juiced carrots count as carbohydrates.

You should eat as many nonstarchy vegetables as you want, varying your selections.

Nonstarchy Vegetables

Amaranth leaves
Arrowhead
Arugula
Asparagus
Balsam-pear
Bamboo shoots
Bean sprouts
Beet greens
Bell peppers
   (red, green, yellow)
Borage
Broadbeans
Broccoli
Brussels sprouts
Butterbur (fuki)
Cabbage
Cardoon
Carrots (raw)
Cassava
Cauliflower
Celeriac
Celery
Celtuce
Chayote fruit
Chicory (witloof)
Chicory greens
Chives
Chrysanthemum
   (garland)
Collard greens
Coriander

Cowpeas (leafy tips)
Cucumber
Dandelion greens
Dock
Eggplant
Endive
Eppaw
Fennel
Gardencress
Garlic
Ginger root
Gourd
Green beans
Hearts of palm
Horseradish-tree,
   leafy tips/pods
Jicama (raw)
Jalapeño peppers
Jew's ear (pepeao)
Jute potherb
Kale
Kohlrabi
Lamb's quarter
Lettuce
Mushrooms
Mustard greens
Nopales
Onions
Parsley
Peppers (sweet green,
   red and yellow)

Pokeberry shoots
Pumpkin flowers/
   leaves
Purslane
Radishes
Radicchio
Salsify
Scallop squash
Sesbania flower
Snap beans
Snow peas
Shallots
Spinach
Spaghetti squash
Summer squash
   (crookneck,
   scallop,
   straight neck,
   zucchini)
Sweet potato leaves
Swiss chard
Taro (leaves or
   shoots)
Tomatoes
Tree fern
Turnip greens
Yardlong bean
Watercress
Waxgourd (Chinese
   preserving melon)

Herbs and Spices

Spices and herbs do not contain sugar or increase insulin secretion. Use them freely.

Healthy Condiments

Balsamic and other vinegars   Natural mustard
Garlic cloves   Olives
Homemade sauces   Peanut sauce (made without sugar)
Low-sodium tamari soy sauce   Salsa (made without sugar)

Some Tips to Remember About Nonstarchy Vegetables

• Do not replace vegetables with vegetable pills. They are a poor substitute for the real food because pills do not alter the glycemic index of your meal. (See chapter 12 for a complete explanation of the glycemic index.)

• Eat fresh (organic, "spray-free") vegetables at every meal—including breakfast.

Carbohydrates

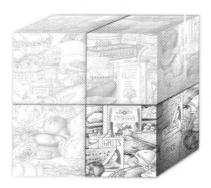

People often ask exactly how many carbohydrates to eat per meal. Everyone needs a different amount of carbohydrates depending on her or his current metabolism and activity level. Think of carbohydrates as fuel. How much fuel do you need at any given moment? If you are going to have an active day, eat more. If you are not very active, eat fewer carbohydrates. But never eat carbohydrates alone. And the quantity you eat must be proportional to your protein and fat intake.

Guideline for Carbohydrate Consumption

Do not count calories, weigh foods or count fat grams. Calculating and focusing on numbers causes an unhealthy obsession with food. However, with carbohydrates the feedback mechanisms occur only after you have overeaten them, so this is the only food group you should be careful with. For a short period of time, you will focus on the numbers. But it does not take long to become educated about the amounts of carbohydrate in the foods you eat; soon it will be automatic. Do not go on a "zero"-gram carbohydrate diet. You may be tempted to because you want to see fast "weight loss," but remember: The first goal is to keep insulin levels balanced. When insulin levels are kept too low (through overexercising and not eating enough food), you will waste away and suffer from depression, fatigue, insomnia and bone loss. This will undermine your goal of achieving optimum health and increasing your metabolism.

Use the following chart to determine how many carbohydrates to eat:

BODY COMPOSITION			Sedentary*	Somewhat Active**	Active***	Extremely Active****	CARBOHYDRATE GRAMS PER MEAL AND SNACK
GUIDELINE FOR CARBOHYDRATE CONSUMPTION **ACTIVITY LEVEL**							
Underweight	Meal		30	30–45	30–60	45–80	
	Snack		0–15	0–15	0–30	0–30	
Normal Body Composition	Meal		30	30–45	30–60	45–75	
	Snack		0–7½	0–7½	0–30	0–30	
Normal Body Composition Fat Around Mid-Section, ("Insulin-Meter")	Meal		15–30	30	30–45	45–60	
	Snack		15	0–7½	0–7½	0–15	
Slightly Overweight with "Insulin-Meter"	Meal		15	15–30	30	45–60	
	Snack		7½–15	0–15	0–15	0–7½	
Overweight with Excessive "Insulin-Meter"	Meal		15	15	15–30	30–45	
	Snack		7½	7½–15	0–15	0–15	

*Sedentary: You do not exercise at all and avoid physical exertion.

**Somewhat Active: You exercise moderately every other day, by bicycling or walking, or engaging in weekend sports such as softball etc., for a total of 2 to 4 hours a week. Or, you are physically active at your job.

***Active: You alternate moderate exercise (2 to 3 times a week) with more rigorous exercise for longer periods of time (1 to 2 times a week) such as aerobics classes, biking, skiing, hiking, jogging, tennis, weight training, for a total of 7 to 10 hours a week.

****Extremely Active: You exercise strenuously 2 to 3 hours every day, engaging in physically challenging competitive sports or activities such as dance, long-distance running, biking, rock climbing, surfing, swimming, weightlifting, for a total of 14 hours or more.

- If you are eating more than 15 grams of carbohydrate per meal, you do not have to eat a snack, unless you are hungry.

- If you are only eating 15 grams of carbohydrate per meal, you must eat two snacks.

- If you have Type II diabetes, eat three meals a day that contain 15 grams of carbohydrate per meal and two 7½-gram carbohydrate snacks.

- If you are depressed and you find yourself getting more depressed, then add 7½ grams carbohydrate per meal and snack.

- If you are losing weight too quickly, feeling sluggish or suffering from insomnia, increase your carbohydrate consumption.

Starchy Vegetables

All items are cooked unless otherwise noted. Each of the following real carbohydrate selections contains fifteen grams of carbohydrate.

Food Item	Serving
Acorn squash	½ cup
Artichokes	1 artichoke
Beets	1 cup
Burdock root (raw)	½ root
Butternut squash	⅔ cup
Carrots	1 cup
Corn	½ cup
Green peas	½ cup
Jerusalem artichokes	½ cup
Leeks	1 cup
Lima beans	½ cup
Lotus root	½ cup
Okra	1 cup
Parsnip	⅔ cup
Potato (baked)	½ medium
Pumpkin	1 cup
Rutabagas (raw)	¼ large
Sweet potato or yam	½ medium
Turnips	½ cup

Legumes

All items are cooked unless otherwise noted. Each of the following real carbohydrate selections contains fifteen grams of carbohydrate.

Food Item	Serving
Adzuki beans	¼ cup
Black beans	⅓ cup
Broadbeans (fava beans)	½ cup
Chickpeas (garbanzo, Bengal)	⅓ cup
Cowpeas (black-eyed peas)	½ cup
Cranberry (Roman) beans	⅓ cup
French beans	⅓ cup
Great Northern beans	⅓ cup
Garbanzo beans	⅓ cup
Hyacinth beans	⅓ cup
Hominy	½ cup
Kidney beans	⅓ cup
Lentils	⅓ cup
Lupins	1 cup
Moth beans	⅓ cup
Mung beans	⅓ cup
Mungo beans (dry)	½ cup
Navy beans	⅓ cup
Pigeon peas	½ cup
Pink beans	⅓ cup
Pinto beans	⅓ cup
Split peas	⅓ cup
White beans	⅓ cup
Yellow beans	⅓ cup

Grains

Always buy grains in their natural state and avoid eating processed grains. Never eat grains that are "flavored" or that have additives such as imitation bacon bits.

Each of the following real carbohydrate selections contains about fifteen grams of carbohydrate.

Food Item (cooked unless noted)	Serving
Barley	⅓ cup
Brown rice	⅓ cup
Buckwheat (whole-grain)	⅓ cup
Buckwheat groats (kasha)	⅓ cup
Bulgur (tabouli)	⅓ cup
Corn bran (crude)	¼ cup
Corn grits, white or yellow	½ cup
Couscous farina	⅓ cup
Millet	⅓ cup
Oats	⅔ cup
Polenta	⅓ cup
Popcorn (popped)[6]	2½ cups
Quinoa	⅓ cup
Rye	¼ cup
Semolina (whole-grain) (dry)	2 tablespoons
Tapioca	¼ cup
Triticale (dry)	2½ tablespoons
Wheat (whole-grain) (dry)	1½ tablespoons
Wheat bran (crude) (dry)	½ cup
Wheat germ (crude) (dry)	⅓ cup
Wild rice	½ cup

---

[6]*Cooking popcorn in hot oil can create trans-fatty acids. The healthiest way to pop popcorn is with a hot air popper, then toss with melted butter.*

Whole-Grain Flour and Meals

Each of the following real carbohydrate selections contains fifteen grams of carbohydrate. All items are dry.

Food Item	Serving
Almond meal	½ cup
Amaranth flour	2 tablespoons
Arrowroot flour	2 tablespoons
Brown rice flour	2 tablespoons
Buckwheat flour (whole-grain)	3½ tablespoons
Carob flour	2½ tablespoons
Corn flour (whole-grain)	2½ tablespoons
Cornmeal	2 tablespoons
Cottonseed flour	1½ ounces
Oat bran flour	⅔ cup
Peanut flour	⅔ cup
Pecan flour	¾ cup
Potato flour	1½ tablespoons
Rye flour	3 tablespoons
Semolina flour (whole-grain)	2 tablespoons
Sesame flour	2½ tablespoons
Soy flour	½ cup
Sunflower seed flour	¾ cup
Semolina (whole-grain)	¼ cup
Sesame flour	1½ ounces
Triticale flour	2½ tablespoons
Whole-wheat flour	3 tablespoons

Be sure to cook with whole-grain flours.

Yogurt

Each of the following real carbohydrate selections contains 15 grams of carbohydrate.

Food Item	Serving
Plain whole milk yogurt	1 cup
Plain whole milk, goat	1 cup
Plain whole milk, Indian buffalo	1 cup
Plain whole milk, sheep	1 cup
Soy	1 cup

Fruit

All fruits are raw, except when noted. Each of the following real carbohydrate selections contains 15 grams of carbohydrate.

Food Item	Serving
Acerola (West Indian cherry)	15 fruits
Apple	1 small
Apples (dried)	3 rings
Applesauce (unsweetened)	¾ cup
Apricots	2 medium
Apricots (dried)	7 halves
Avocados (California)	1 avocado
Avocados (Florida)	½ avocado
Bananas	½ medium
Bananas (dehydrated)	1 tablespoon
Blackberries	¾ cup
Blueberries	¾ cup
Boysenberries	1 cup
Breadfruit	⅛ small
Carambola (starfruit)	1½ cups (sliced)
Cherimoya (custard apple)	2 ounces
Cherries	1 cup (with pits)
Crabapples	¾ cup (sliced)
Cranberries (unsweetened)	1 cup, whole
Currants (European, fresh)	1 cup
Currants (red or white)	1 cup
Currants (Zante, dried)	2 tablespoons
Dates	2 medium
Elderberries	½ cup
Figs	2 medium
Figs (dried)	1 medium
Gooseberries	1 cup

Grapefruit	½ large
Grapes (American)	15 grapes
Grapes (European)	7 grapes
Groundcherries (cape-gooseberries)	1 cup
Guavas (common)	1½ fruit
Guavas (strawberry)	15 guavas
Jackfruit	2 ounces
Java-plum (Jambolan)	¾ cup
Jujube	¼ cup
Jujube (dried)	1 tablespoon
Kiwi fruit (Chinese gooseberries)	1 large
Kumquats	5 kumquats
Lemons	3 medium
Limes	2 medium
Litchis	7 fruits
Litchis (dried)	2 tablespoons
Loganberries	¾ cup
Longans	31 fruits
Longans (dried)	2 tablespoons
Loquats	5 large
Mammey-apple	1 medium
Mangos	½ medium
Melons (cantaloupe)	1 cup (cubes)
Melons (casaba)	1½ cup (cubes)
Melons (honeydew)	1 cup (diced)
Mulberries	1 cup
Nectarines	1 medium
Oranges	1 medium
Tangerines	2 small
Papayas	½ cup (mashed)
Passion fruit (granadilla)	3 fruits
Peaches	1 medium
Peaches (dried)	2 halves
Pears	½ large

Pears (dried)	1 half
Persimmons (Japanese)	½ medium
Persimmons (Japanese, dried)	½ medium
Persimmons (native)	2 medium
Pineapple	¾ cup
Plantains (cooked)	⅓ cup
Plums	2 fruits
Pomegranates (Chinese apple)	½ fruit
Prickly pears	1½ medium
Prunes	3 prunes
Pomelo	¾ cup
Quinces	1 medium
Raisins (dark/golden seedless)	2 tablespoons
Raspberries	1 cup
Rhubarb	7 stalks
Rose-apples	2 medium
Sapotes (marmalade plum)	½ medium
Soursop (guanabana)	½ cup
Strawberries	1½ cup
Sugar-apples (sweetsop)	½ fruit
Sun-dried tomatoes	1/6 ounce
Tamarinds	15 fruits
Tomatoes (green and red)	1 medium
Tomatillos	1 large
Watermelon	1¼ cup (diced)

Eat fruits in their natural state. Do not eat fruit cocktail or fruits canned in syrup. Eat organic, "spray-free" fruits.

Man-Made Carbohydrate Options

I do not advise eating man-made carbohydrates. But for the sake of convenience, some man-made carbohydrates are better than others. Each of these man-made carbohydrate selections contains 15 grams of carbohydrates. *Remember, you should eat real carbohydrates whenever possible. Fresh-baked bread is preferable because it contains no additives.*

Bread

Food Item	Serving
Bread crumbs	1½ tablespoons
Corn tortilla	1 medium tortilla
Cracked-wheat bread	1 slice
Cracker meal	1½ tablespoons
Low-carbohydrate bread[7]	2 slices
Oat bran bread	1 slice
Oatmeal bread	1 slice
Pumpernickel bread	1 regular slice
Rice bran bread	1 slice
Rye bread	1 large slice
Wheat bran bread	1 slice
Wheat germ bread	1 slice
Wheatberry	1 slice
Whole-grain hamburger/hot-dog bun	½ bun
Whole-grain raisin bread	1 slice
Whole-wheat English muffins	½ muffin
Whole-grain dinner roll	1 roll
Whole-grain pita	1 small pita
Whole-grain, 7-grain bread	1 slice

[7] *Any bread that contains 7½ grams of carbohydrate or less.*

Crackers

Most crackers contain many additives, including hydrogenated fats. Look for crackers that are low-carbohydrate, whole-grain and do not contain hydrogenated fats. Each selection below contains 15 grams of carbohydrate.

Food Item	Serving
Rice crackers	4 crackers
Rice cakes	2 cakes
Rye crispbread	2 crackers
Rye wafers (Wasa)	2 crackers
Rusk toast	1½ ounces
Wheat crackers (AK-Mak)	4 crackers
Wheat Euphrates	5 crackers
Wheat melba toast	3 toasts
Whole-wheat Matzo	½ (6"x 4")

Liquid Carbohydrates

Liquid carbohydrates are digested and absorbed faster than solid carbohydrates, which translates to a higher glycemic index and therefore a higher insulin-to-glucagon ratio. For example, a four-ounce glass of milk has a higher glycemic index than one slice of whole-grain bread, although they both contain fifteen grams of carbohydrate, because a liquid carbohydrate can be digested and absorbed faster than bread. So the milk acts all at once to bring insulin levels higher.

Fruit juice, though natural, is mostly sugar water. One glass of orange juice is approximately three oranges, minus the benefits of fiber—and the glycemic index is much higher than in fruit. If you must drink fruit juice, dilute it four to one.

The human body is composed of 50 to 60 percent water. Fluid balance is a necessity for true health. There is no substitute for drinking water. Drink eight to ten eight-ounce glasses per day.

The following are a few juices that are good for you. Each selection contains the glycemic index equivalent of 15 grams of carbohydrate.

Food Item	Serving
Carrot	3 fluid ounces
Vegetable	6 fluid ounces
Tomato	6 fluid ounces

Some Tips to Remember About Carbohydrates

• When you eat an excess of carbohydrates, insulin levels rise.

• Your body does not regulate the amount of carbohydrates you eat, as it does with protein and fats. You will eventually feel satiated, but not until you have already overeaten carbohydrates.

• Choose between fifteen and eighty grams of carbohydrate per meal, depending on your physical condition and metabolism and immediate energy needs.

• If you are only eating fifteen grams of carbohydrate per meal, you must eat five meals per day.

• Always eat carbohydrates with protein and fats.

• If you eat more carbohydrates than are needed, the excess will be converted into fats and stored in the fat cells.

• Vary your selections of carbohydrates from meal to meal and day to day.

• Eat whole grains, legumes, starchy vegetables and fruits. Avoid man-made carbohydrates.

• Do not decrease your caloric intake as you decrease your carbohydrate intake. Decreasing calories leads to the shutting down of your metabolism.

Vitamins and Minerals

The best way to get vitamins and minerals is from their natural state in real, whole foods grown in vitamin- and mineral-rich soil. If you feel you need to supplement your diet, take a multivitamin supplement. If you are serotonin depleted (see chapter 4 for low-serotonin symptoms), I recommend balanced nutrition and hormone replacement therapy, as needed. I also prescribe: a well-balanced multivitamin; a stress B complex with breakfast; 250 to 300 milligrams of St. John's wort in the morning (slowly increase to 250 to 300 milligrams three times a day, as needed); 1,000 milligrams twice a day of essential fatty acids (capsule or liquid); 250 to 500 milligrams of L-tryptophan (available by prescription only), or 25 to 50 milligrams of 5-hydroxytryptophan (5-HTP) (available over-the-counter) at bedtime; and 250 to 500 milligrams of magnesium and 1,000 milligrams of calcium at bedtime.[8]

The following is a list of some important vitamins and minerals and the foods that contain them:

Calcium is a mineral found in salmon, sardines, chicken, navy beans, milk, cheeses, broccoli, turnip greens and tofu. A common misconception is that calcium is important only for bones and teeth. But a deficiency leads to deterioration of bone and teeth because the body uses calcium from these stores for its more important roles in the rest of the body, such as blood clotting, muscle locomotion, transmission of nerve impulses, activation of enzymes and hormone secretion.

Carnitine is found in animal products, especially red meat. The highest concentration is in liver, lamb and beef. This lipoprotein is essential to the transport of long-chain fatty acids and the transport

---

[8] *If you take too much magnesium you may have loose bowel movements. If this happens, decrease your dose.*

of vitamins E and C. A lack of carnitine in the diet leads to low HDL levels, high serum cholesterol and triglyceride levels, and an overall difficulty in losing body fat.

Chromium is a mineral found in meats, cheese, eggs and whole grains. Chromium is important in sugar metabolism. Chromium deficiency leads to insulin resistance, higher serum triglycerides and cholesterol levels, lower HDL levels and heart disease.

Cyanocobalamin (B$_{12}$) is a vitamin found in animal and animal-derived foods such as liver, meat, saltwater fish, oysters, eggs and milk. B$_{12}$ is essential to the normal function of all body cells and the growth of red blood cells. B$_{12}$ deficiency can result in anemia and nerve cell damage.

Folate is an essential vitamin found in liver, beef, fish, green leafy vegetables, asparagus, broccoli, dry beans, lentils and whole grains. Folate is essential in the metabolism of homocysteine (an amino acid), in the maturation of red blood cells and in the normal functioning of all body cells. Folate deficiency results in nontropical sprue, with symptoms of weakness, decreased hunger, gas, loose stools and malabsorption of food.

Magnesium is a mineral found primarily in beans, broccoli, avocados and figs. Magnesium helps with muscle relaxation and energy release and is a catalyst for important metabolic reactions. Magnesium is a coenzyme to help your body build proteins and produce serotonin. Magnesium prevents constipation. A deficiency leads to muscle spasms, nervousness, irritability and tremors.

Niacin (B$_3$) is a vitamin present in meat, fish, poultry, liver, eggs, legumes, mushrooms and whole grains. Niacin deficiency results in dry skin, decreased energy and loose stools.

Pyridoxine (B$_6$) is a vitamin found in legumes, seeds, whole grains, corn, potatoes, green leafy vegetables and green beans. It helps with sugar and protein metabolism as well as the production of serotonin. Pyridoxine deficiency can be the cause of anemia, fatigue, PMS and a low-serotonin state.

Riboflavin (B₂) is a vitamin found in meat, fish, eggs, liver, milk and green leafy vegetables. This vitamin is involved in protein metabolism and eye function. People lacking in riboflavin can experience dry, itchy skin and sensitivity to light.

Thiamine (B₁) is found in chicken, liver, fish, pork, beef, nuts, lentils, whole grains and potatoes. It helps with stored sugar utilization and is important in the metabolism and the maintenance of the brain. A deficiency in this vitamin can result in loss of appetite, hard infrequent stools, irritability and lethargy.

Vitamin A is found in foods of both animal and plant origin, such as beef, liver, dandelion greens, sweet potatoes, apricots, pumpkin, spinach and butter. It is important for healthy vision and healthy skin. If left uncorrected, vitamin A deficiency can lead to poor night vision and blindness as well as skin breakdowns, which make it easier for bacteria to enter the body, leading to increased infections.

Vitamin C is found in cabbage, kale, parsley, turnip greens, broccoli, tomatoes, citrus fruits, strawberries and cantaloupe. Vitamin C helps heal wounds and broken bones, promotes tooth and bone growth, protects against heart disease, increases iron absorption and helps with collagen formation. Deficiency can lead to inflammation of the gums, slow wound healing, anemia, scurvy and increased bruising.

Vitamin E is found in egg yolks, green leafy vegetables, vegetable oils, whole grains and legumes. Vitamin E is an important antioxidant. It also helps stabilize all cell membranes and is important in blood-cell formation. A deficiency in this vitamin can result in abnormal fat deposits, red blood cell disintegration and cellular oxidation (one of the processes that leads to arterial plaque).

Vitamin and mineral deficiencies are caused by stress, caffeine, alcohol, aspartame, tobacco, steroids and poor nutrition.

As you now know, many substances will put you on the accelerated metabolic aging track. Chapter 26 details what you should avoid eating.

Twenty-Six

What Not to Eat

Damaged Fats

I have heard people say, "Oh, you're the doctor who tells people to eat hamburgers and french fries!" Once you have read this book cover to cover, you will know that I *never* recommend french fries or any other foods prepared with damaged fats. Diets of french fries, doughnuts and other items made with damaged fats have contributed to the rise in disease over the past twenty years. Fats in nature are good, but what we have done to good natural fats—deep-frying and processing them from their natural state into oils—damages human physiology.

I am very concerned when I hear that a patient is eating fried foods, margarine or other damaged fats because the cells of the body cannot recognize and metabolize any of these. Instead, damaged fat molecules become cellular debris, clogging cellular compartments and, in turn, damaging those cells. This contributes to the accelerated metabolic aging process.

Damaged fats fall into three categories:

• Trans-fatty acids

• Oxidized

• Hydrogenated

Trans-fatty Acids

Over the last few years, the term "trans-fatty acids" has been thrown around. And most people have learned that trans-fatty acids are unhealthy. But most do not know what a trans-fatty acid is.

In nature, fats occur in the "cis" molecular configuration. "Cis" means the same side. When the hydrogen atoms around the double bond are found on the same side as the carbon atoms, they are said to be in the "cis" configuration. Since this is the form in which they are found in nature, the "cis" configuration is desirable.

You have heard that polyunsaturated foods are good for you. This is true of polyunsaturated *fats* that are eaten in their natural state, such as nuts and seeds, salmon and other fish, soybeans, corn and essential fatty acids. However, most polyunsaturated *oils* are not good for you because they are processed out of their natural state by using very high temperatures (for example, corn oil removed from corn). This process changes the natural "cis" configuration to an unhealthy "trans" configuration. "Trans" means the hydrogen atoms are now on opposite sides of the carbon double bond. Unfortunately, during processing a good percentage of the "cis" molecules turn to "trans," and this is not a good thing for the human body because we do not have the enzyme necessary to fully metabolize the transfat into energy. When you eat trans-fatty acids, you end up with debris that clogs your cells, contributing to accelerated metabolic aging.

It is not healthy to eat any polyunsaturated oil that has been extracted from its natural source by using a heat process. But it is even worse to cook with this type of damaged fat. Because polyunsaturated oils are easily damaged under heat, cooking with them compounds the damage by converting yet more "cis" to "trans" configurations. Even though saturated fats are much more stable under heat, and therefore healthier to cook with, current thought is that polyunsaturated fats are healthier. Fast-food chains have reacted to the misguided fear of saturated oils by switching to polyunsaturated oils for cooking, which means that people are eating even *more* trans-fatty acids. While fast-food franchises have met the demands of the public by switching from saturated oils to polyunsaturated oils, they are only further contributing to the decline in people's health.

Cis Configuration

$$- \overset{|}{\underset{|}{C}} - \overset{\overset{H}{|}}{C} = \overset{\overset{H}{|}}{C} - \overset{|}{\underset{|}{C}} - \overset{|}{\underset{|}{C}} -$$

Hydrogen molecules are on same side

Trans Configuration

$$- \overset{|}{\underset{|}{C}} - \overset{\overset{H}{|}}{\underset{|}{C}} = \overset{|}{\underset{\underset{H}{|}}{C}} - \overset{|}{\underset{|}{C}} - \overset{|}{\underset{|}{C}} -$$

Hydrogen molecules are on opposite side

Because polyunsaturated oils are damaged during processing and cooking at high temperatures, you are better off using and cooking with saturated or monounsaturated oils. Avoid these polyunsaturated oils (unless they are pure-pressed; then you can use them for salad dressing but not for cooking).

Corn oil	Safflower oil	Sunflower oil
Cottonseed oil	Sesame oil	Walnut oil
Poppyseed oil	Soybean oil	

Oxidation

Another way oils become damaged is through exposure to air. The oxygen in the air binds to the carbon atom where the hydrogen atom is missing (the double-bonded carbons) and steals an electron from the fat molecule. The fat that is now missing an electron is damaged, or "oxidized." Oxidized fats are free radicals. (See page 32 for free radicals.)

Oxidation can be seen visually as rancid fats. When butter turns dark yellow or oils go brown, they are rancid. Rancid fats should never be eaten. Oxidation occurs more easily to fats that are removed from their natural source (e.g., corn oil taken out of corn). This is because oils are found in their natural source together with antioxidants such as lecithin and vitamin E, both of which are removed or destroyed during the refining process. Oxidation also occurs more easily at higher temperatures. *All fats should be refrigerated to prevent oxidation.*

Hydrogenated Fats

Other terms you may be familiar with are hydrogenated and partially hydrogenated fats. These are created when natural polyunsaturated oil has been altered by a chemical process that adds hydrogen molecules to the fat molecule. This process changes naturally occurring oils, which are liquid at room temperature, into solid fats. This is how margarine is made from corn oil, for example. From the fat molecules the hydrogenation process creates new chemical structures as well as those unwanted trans-fatty acids. Margarine and shortening are two of the most damaging fatty substances you can eat because they also contribute to accelerated metabolic aging.

General Guidelines for Avoiding Damaged Fats

Whenever possible, eat all fats, fatty foods and oils without cooking them. Unfortunately, eating raw foods such as meat and eggs poses serious health problems, such as the possibility of acquiring deadly bacterial infections. For that reason, the way foods are cooked becomes the issue. Never overcharbroil—blacken the outside of the meat—because this damages the fat in the meat. Leaner meats are best because they do not contain extra fat that can be damaged by cooking. It is best to cook at slow, low temperatures rather than at higher temperatures. Medium rare is healthier than well done.

Some Tips to Remember About Damaged Fats

- The only bad fats are man-made and damaged fats.

- Do not eat processed fats or foods made with processed fats.

- Saturated and monounsaturated fats are more resistant to damage from heat, and can be used for cooking.

- Polyunsaturated fats found in their natural state are healthy. Polyunsaturated fats processed into oils and/or used for cooking are not healthy.

- Never deep-fry foods.

- Eat fresh fats and keep fats refrigerated to prevent rancidity.

- Avoid all hydrogenated and partially hydrogenated oils.

- Cook fatty meats at low, even temperatures to avoid damaging fats.

Avoid Fats That Contain Damaged Fats, Chemicals and/or Sugar

Bottled salad dressings
Buttermilk
Coconut oil
Cream substitutes
Cream containing chemicals
Deep-fat-fried foods
Half-and-half
High-fat meats that have been
   cooked at high temperatures
Hydrogenated oils
Imitation mayonnaise

Imitation sour cream
Lard/shortening
Margarine
Non-dairy creamers
Palm oil
Pressurized whipped cream
   and dessert toppings
Processed foods and fast
   foods using hydrogenated oils
Rancid fats
Sandwich spreads

Other Unhealthy Items to Avoid

Do Not Eat Processed and High-Sodium Sausages

Barbecue loaf
Beer salami
Beerwurst
Beerwurst salami
Bologna
Corned beef loaf

Honey loaf
Honey-roll sausage
Lebanon bologna
Luxury loaf
Mother's loaf
Pastrami

Peppered loaf
Pepperoni
Picnic loaf
Pork headcheese
Salami
Vienna sausage

Do Not Eat Man-Made or Refined Grain Products

Bagels
Banana bread
Biscuits
Bread sticks
Bread stuffing
Chinese noodles
Cold cereal
Corn cakes
Cornbread*
Cornbread stuffing
Cream of rice*
Cream of wheat*
Croissants*
Croutons

Crumpets
Dinner rolls
Egg bread
Flour tortilla
French bread
Ice cream cone
Irish soda bread
Italian bread
Macaroni
Muffins
Navajo bread
Noodles
Pancakes
Pasta

Phyllo dough
Pie crust
Pizza dough
Popovers
Puff pastry
Scones
Sourdough bread*
Spaghetti
Waffles
White English muffins
White hamburger and
    hot-dog buns
White rice
Wonton wrappers

Do Not Eat Sugar and Desserts

Banana chips
Brown sugar
Cakes
Candy
Caramel or other
    flavored popcorn
Cheesecake
Cocoa
Coffeecake
Cookies
Dessert toppings
Doughnuts
Eclairs
Frosting
Frozen desserts

Fruit butters
Fruit leathers
Gelatin desserts
Granola and other
    snack bars
Honey*
Ice cream
Jams, jellies, pre-
    serves, marmalade
Milk shakes
Molasses
Pastries
Pie
Protein bars (with
    man-made chemicals)

Processed yogurt
    (low-fat, non-fat
    or flavored yogurt)
Pudding
Sherbet
Strudel
Sweet rolls
Syrups (fudge,
    corn, high-fructose
    corn, malt, maple,
    sorghum, butter-
    scotch or caramel)
Toaster pastries
White sugar

*Eat these foods in moderation.

Do Not Eat Processed Snack Foods

Beef jerky	Pork skins	Tortilla chips*
Corn chips	Potato chips	Trail mix packaged
Corn nuts*	Pretzels	with chocolate chips
Meat-based sticks	Sesame sticks	and other sweets
Pizza†	Taro chips*	

Do Not Eat Processed Foods

Canned foods	Mixes	Packaged foods
Dried soups	Fast foods	

Do Not Eat Condiments
(They Contain Sugar and Chemical Additives)

Barbecue sauces	Ketchup	Relishes
Fish sauces	Meat extender	Sweet pickles
Gravies	Meat tenderizer	Worcestershire
Hoisin sauce	Oyster sauce	

*Eat these foods in moderation, and only when prepared with pure-pressed mono-unsaturated oil.
†You can eat sauceless thin-crust pizza or thin-crust pizza made with sugarless sauce.

Other Substances to Avoid

Alcohol: Alcohol is derived from grain or fruit, which are carbohydrates. Because alcohol is toxic to cells and increases insulin levels, drinking alcohol accelerates the metabolic aging process. Recent studies have also linked alcohol consumption to breast cancer.

Aspartame: Aspartame can lead to carbohydrate craving. Aspartame breaks down into methyl alcohol, a chemical that is poisonous to the human body. Aspartame is known to cause headaches, dizziness, anxiety, depression, memory loss, confusion, vision loss and convulsive seizures.

Caffeine: Caffeine is a stimulant. All stimulants can cause insulin resistance and therefore increase the accelerated metabolic aging process. All stimulants are eventually depressants because they deplete serotonin. If you must drink coffee, drink water-processed, decaffeinated coffee and put whole cream in it, which contains no carbohydrates. Both milk and half-and-half contain carbohydrates.

High Fructose Corn Syrup: Fructose occurs naturally in corn and fruit. Studies have proven that fructose is more damaging to cells than sucrose (table sugar). High-fructose corn syrup is concentrated fructose that is used to sweeten processed foods. It is much more damaging than the fructose found in natural foods. Eating foods containing high-fructose corn syrup also leads to carbohydrate craving. Beverages containing sugar, high-fructose corn sweeteners and sugar substitutes deplete you of vitamins and minerals and lead to cellular dehydration. High-fructose corn syrup contributes to the accelerated metabolic aging process more than any other form of sugar.

Olestra (Olean): Olestra interferes with the body's absorption of fat and fat-soluble vitamins. Never eat anything containing Olestra.

Refined and Processed Foods: Refined carbohydrates (white rice, white flour, cereals and so on) are not whole foods. Taking the "wholeness" out of a carbohydrate throws off the balance of foods. Carbohydrates are burned for energy with the aid of enzymes that are helped by the B vitamins. The more carbohydrates you eat, the more B vitamins you need. At the same time, eating carbohydrates depletes B vitamins.

Saccharin: Saccharin is an invented substance and contributes to the accelerated metabolic aging process.

Salt: Do not add salt to your foods. Foods contain sufficient salt for bodily functions. Your body strives to maintain a salt balance, so extra salt puts stress on your kidneys to eliminate it.

Sucrose (White Sugar), Fructose, Maltose, Dextrose, Polydextrose, Corn Syrup, Molasses, Sorbital, Maltodextrin: Sugar causes multiple vitamin and mineral deficiencies and prolonged high insulin levels, which contribute to the accelerated metabolic aging process.

Tobacco: The hydrocarbons in tobacco damage cells; nicotine is a stimulant. The nicotine in tobacco causes insulin resistance and increases blood pressure and heart rate. Medical studies have confirmed that smokers have an increased risk of developing Type II diabetes, lung cancer, osteoporosis, emphysema and heart disease. Tobacco is an oxidant that damages cholesterol, as well as brain and body cells.

Do Not Eat Fast Foods

Since fast foods are processed, and contain additives and damaged fats, they contribute to the accelerated metabolic aging process. Below is a sampling of the sugars, salts, carcinogens, chemicals and trans-fatty acids contained in fast foods.

Chicken Fajita (meat portion): Lactose, salt, hydrolyzed corn gluten, soy and wheat gluten proteins, autolyzed yeast (contains MSG), maltodextrin, soy sauce solids, modified corn starch, partially hydrogenated soybean and cottonseed oil, dextrose, lactic acid and silicon dioxide.

Chicken Filet: Sugar, soy sauce powder, dehydrated sherry wine (maltodextrin added), salt, carrageenan gum, partially hydrogenated soybean and cottonseed oils, disodium inosinate and disodium guanylate, and sodium phosphate.

Bleu Cheese Dressing: Corn syrup, maltodextrin, high-fructose corn syrup, xanthan gum, color, propylene glycol alginate, fumaric acid, potassium sorbate, disodium EDTA, BHT, disodium inosinate and disodium guanylate.

The FDA Total Diet Study found that fast-food hamburgers, across the board, contained 113 different pesticide residues. Fast-food hamburgers are also a source of trans-fatty acids.

Bacon Cheeseburger:

Bacon: Bacon cured with salt, sugar, smoke flavor, sodium phosphates, sodium erythorbate, sodium nitrate.

American Cheese: Sodium citrate, modified cheese, sodium phosphate, salt, sorbic acid, acetic acid, phosphoric acid, artificial colors.

Hamburger Bun: Corn syrup, mono- and diglycerides, sodium stearoyl lactylate, polysorbate 60, calcium iodate, wheat gluten.

Not only are fast foods a source of refined sugar, chemicals and damaged fats, but they also contain many carbohydrates. Below are some typical selections of carbohydrates (in grams) from popular fast-food restaurants:

Bacon cheeseburger: 59 grams

Baked potato with broccoli and cheese: 90 grams

Bran muffin: 61 grams

Chicken teriyaki bowl: 115 grams

Coleslaw: 21 grams (from added sugar)

Crosscut-fries: 55 grams

Egg rolls: 92 grams

Garden rice: 23 grams

Hot & spicy chicken breast: 23 grams (from breading alone)

Light chicken burrito: 62 grams

Low-fat milk: 12 grams, but acts more like 24 grams

Orange juice: 20 grams, but acts more like 30 to 40 grams

Root beer: 61 grams but acts more like 80 to 100 grams

Small lemonade: 24 grams, but acts more like 30 to 40 grams

Taco salad: 53 grams

Everyone has busy schedules, and fast foods, TV or microwavable dinners, and processed foods have become part of life. But you will find that you can roast a chicken and make a salad in a very short time, and with some practice you can prepare easy meals made with real foods that are less expensive than processed foods. Chapter 27 offers four weeks of meat-based meal plans and four weeks of vegetarian meal plans to get you started.

Twenty-Seven

Planning Your Meals

Eating a variety of foods is the best way to achieve balance. The ideal is to eat only carbohydrates found in nature—anything that you could (at least, in theory) pick, gather or milk—such as potatoes, whole-grain rice, peas, corn, lima beans and fruits. But this is not always possible. You will see in the menu plans that breads are included; however, processed grain-based products should not be eaten regularly. When you are going to eat them, choose whole grains (which are different from whole wheat, which is a more processed bread). Look for products that are the least processed.

A vital ingredient to good eating is enjoyment. Sauces made with cream and butter, creamy salad dressings and good oils add flavor to meals. There are many good cookbooks available containing balanced recipes. Like Sarah, whom you read about in chapter 22, my patients tell me that they are once again using cookbooks they had put away during their years of low-fat dieting. *The Schwarzbein Principle Cookbook* and *The Schwarzbein Principle Vegetarian Cookbook* are both combined specifically for enjoyment and balanced nutrition by "*The Schwarzbein Principle* Chef" Evelyn Jacob Jaffe.

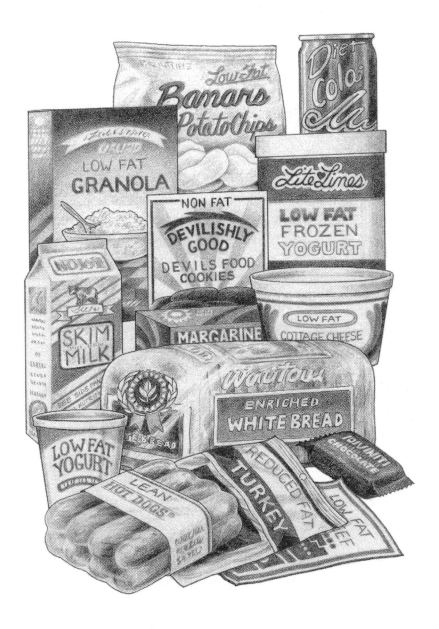

Figure 27-1. What Your Groceries Used to Look Like

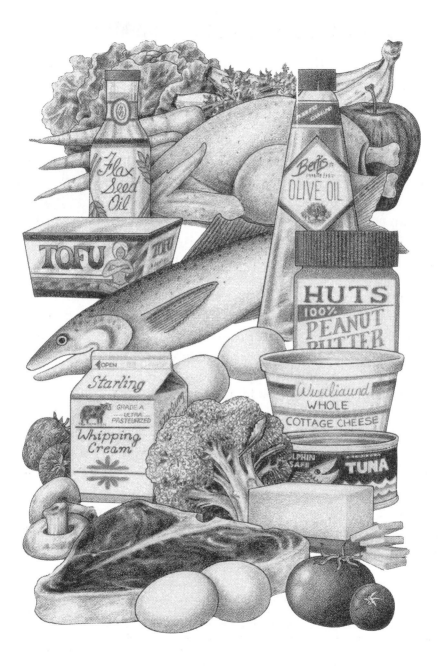

**Figure 27-2. What Your Groceries Look Like
on the Schwarzbein Program**

Four Weeks of Healing Program Meal Plans

The meal plans that follow are designed specifically for those who are on the healing program. Each daily menu consists of three meals containing approximately 15 grams of carbohydrate, each with two approximately 7½-gram carbohydrate snacks. Carbohydrates are the only food group that you need to restrict. There are no amounts specified for proteins, fats and nonstarchy vegetables. Eat as much of these foods as you need, keeping your meal balanced. A good way of gauging this is to see that the protein, fat and nonstarchy vegetables are equal in portion size on your plate. However, if you find that you are too full to eat snacks, you should eat less at meals. If you are too hungry between meals, you should eat more protein, fats and nonstarchy vegetables. The healing program is not meant to continue for the rest of your life. Once your symptoms or illnesses are corrected, you must increase carbohydrate consumption to meet your increased metabolic needs. Please refer to the Guideline for Carbohydrate Consumption on page 260 to see if the Healing Program is right for you. If you require more carbohydrates per meal and snacks, you can still use these meal plans by simply adding carbohydrates.[1]

These meal plans have been designed to help you understand how to create balanced meals. It is not necessary to follow these menus rigidly. Find the meals and snacks you like and mix and match. The goal is to ultimately understand how to select and balance foods whether cooking at home or eating in a restaurant.[2]

Included in these meal plans are a selection of recipes excerpted from *The Schwarzbein Principle Cookbook* and *The Schwarzbein Principle Vegetarian Cookbook*.

---

[1] *These meal plans are designed to keep your insulin-to-glucagon ratio and your glycemic index balanced (see page 122) by providing 15 grams of carbohydrate per balanced meal. While many foods contain some carbohydrate, such as tofu, they are also high in protein, fat, or fiber, and, if eaten alone, would result in a balanced insulin-to-glucagon ratio and glycemic index. It is only necessary to restrict those foods that, if they were eaten alone, would cause a rapid rise in insulin resulting in an imbalanced insulin-to-glucagon ratio and glycemic index. For that reason, only the foods that are italized are considered to contain the 15 grams of carbohydrate allowed per meal on the healing program.*

[2] *All nuts should be raw, dry-roasted or roasted in peanut oil. You can substitute cheese with any other white cheese (see cheese list on page 246).*

Day 1

Breakfast: Scrambled eggs with nitrate-free sausages. ⅔ cup *oatmeal* with butter and cream. Sliced tomatoes.

Snack: ¼ cup *sunflower seeds*.

Lunch: Cobb salad (made with chopped chicken, nitrate-free bacon, hard-boiled egg, bleu cheese, salad greens and tomatoes). Olive-oil-and-vinegar dressing. 1 small *apple*.

Snack: ¼ cup *almonds*. String cheese.

Dinner: Roast pork loin. ⅓ cup *brown rice* with butter. Asparagus with butter. Mixed-greens salad with tomatoes and cucumbers, tossed with olive-oil-and-vinegar dressing.

Day 2

Breakfast: Annette Matrisciano's Cheesy Eggs (see recipe, page 322). 1 slice buttered low-carbohydrate *toast*. 3 ounces *vegetable juice*.

Snack: 2 tablespoons *peanut butter* on celery sticks.

Lunch: Salade Niçoise (see recipe, page 329). 1 large or 2 small *tangerines*.

Snack: ⅓ cup *hummus* with carrot, bell pepper and celery sticks.

Dinner: Broiled chicken breasts. Buttered green beans. ¼ cup mashed *potatoes* with butter. Lettuce, cucumber and tomato salad tossed with olive-oil-and-vinegar dressing. ½ cup fresh *raspberries* with unsweetened whipping cream.

Day 3

Breakfast: Spinach and feta-cheese omelet. 1 cup cubed *honeydew melon*.

Snack: Turkey and Swiss cheese. 1 tablespoon *raisins*.

Lunch: Tuna salad (made with tuna, diced celery and mayonnaise topped with ½ *avocado* and sliced tomato). Carrot sticks.

Snack: 1½ tablespoons *cashew butter* on celery sticks.

Dinner: Steak fajitas (made with onion, bell peppers, grated Monterey Jack cheese, tomato, lettuce and sour cream.) 1 *corn tortilla*.

Day 4

Breakfast: Spicy Chicken Frittata (see recipe, page 326). ½ cup *grits* with butter and cream.

Snack: Mozzarella cheese. 2 low-carbohydrate *whole-grain crackers*.

Lunch: Seafood salad (made with shrimp, crab and hard-boiled eggs) on bed of mixed greens, tomatoes and cucumbers tossed with olive-oil-and-vinegar dressing. ¾ cup fresh cubed *pineapple*.

Snack: 1 cup *cottage cheese*. Carrot sticks.

Dinner: Roast beef. ½ *baked potato* with butter, sour cream and chives. Mixed vegetables with butter. Green salad with tomatoes and cucumbers tossed with olive-oil-and-vinegar dressing.

Day 5

Breakfast: Nancy Deville's Crustless Spinach and Mushroom Quiche (see recipe, page 323). ½ cup *oatmeal* with butter and unsweetened cream.

Snack: String cheese. ½ small *apple*.

Lunch: Turkey breast sandwich with mayonnaise on ½ *whole-grain roll*. Lettuce and tomato salad tossed with olive-oil-and-vinegar dressing.

Snack: Deviled eggs. ½ medium *orange*.

Dinner: Broiled fish of your choice. ½ medium roasted *sweet potato* with butter. Steamed broccoli with butter. Mixed-greens salad tossed with sesame-oil-and-lime-juice dressing. ¾ cup cubed *watermelon*.

Day 6

Breakfast: Cream cheese, spinach and mushroom omelet. 1 slice buttered *whole-grain toast* or 2 slices buttered low-carbohydrate *toast*.

Snack: Ham and Swiss cheese. 1 *fig*.

Lunch: Chicken salad (made with diced chicken, sour cream and mayonnaise) over bed of greens with mushrooms, cucumber, tomato and sprouts tossed with olive-oil-and-vinegar dressing. 1 medium *nectarine*.

Snack: ½ cup *cottage cheese*. ¼ cup unsweetened *applesauce*.

Dinner: Pork chops. ¼ cup *lima beans*. Coleslaw (made with shredded cabbage, carrots and onions with mayonnaise-and-vinegar dressing). ½ cup fresh *strawberries* topped with unsweetened whipping cream.

Day 7

Breakfast: San Francisco Joe's Special (see recipe, page 324).
1 medium *orange*.

Snack: Swiss cheese. ½ small *apple*.

Lunch: Grilled nitrate-free ham and Monterey Jack or Gruyère sandwich on 2 slices low-carbohydrate *bread*. Carrot sticks.

Snack: ¼ cup *cashews*.

Dinner: Broiled chicken breasts. ⅓ cup *kasha*. Steamed broccoli with butter and Parmesan cheese. Mixed-greens salad tossed with olive-oil-and-vinegar dressing.

Day 8

Breakfast: Spinach and mushroom omelet. 1 cup cubed *cantaloupe*.

Snack: ½ serving *Tofu "Egg" Salad* (see recipe, page 330). Carrot sticks.

Lunch: Chef's salad (made with roast beef, Swiss cheese, hard-boiled eggs, salad greens and tomatoes tossed with olive-oil-and-vinegar dressing). ½ buttered *whole-grain roll*.

Snack: ⅓ cup *hummus* with carrot and celery sticks.

Dinner: Barbecued spareribs (do not use sweetened or bottled barbecue sauce). ½ *baked potato* with butter, sour cream and chives. Mixed-greens salad tossed with olive-oil-and-lemon-juice dressing.

Day 9

Breakfast: Poached eggs. ½ buttered, toasted *English muffin*. Sliced tomatoes.

Snack: String cheese. ¾ cup sliced *strawberries* with unsweetened whipping cream.

Lunch: Turkey patties. ½ cup *cottage cheese*. Sliced tomatoes. ½ cup cubed *honeydew melon*.

Snack: Swiss cheese. ¼ cup *almonds*.

Dinner: Greek-Style Baked Fish (see recipe, page 335). ⅓ cup *brown rice* with butter. Mixed-greens salad tossed with olive-oil-and-vinegar dressing.

Day 10

Breakfast: Scrambled eggs with ham, onions and bell pepper. ¼ cup roasted *potatoes*.

Snack: 4 tablespoons *almond butter* on celery sticks.

Lunch: Beef stew (limit carbohydrate portion to ¼ cup *carrots* and ¼ cup *potatoes*). ¼ cup *boysenberries* with unsweetened whipping cream.

Snack: Mozzarella cheese. ½ cup *cherries*.

Dinner: Roasted turkey breast. Brussels sprouts with butter. ½ cup *acorn squash* with butter. Mixed-greens salad tossed with olive-oil-and-vinegar dressing.

Day 11

Breakfast: Three-minute eggs. 1 slice buttered *whole-grain toast*, or 2 slices buttered low-carbohydrate *toast*. 3 ounces *vegetable juice*.

Snack: Buffalo mozzarella cheese. ½ *peach*.

Lunch: Nitrate-free chicken hot dogs on ½ *whole-grain bun* with mayonnaise and mustard. Coleslaw (made with shredded cabbage, carrots and onions with mayonnaise-and-vinegar dressing).

Snack: ⅓ cup *hummus* on celery sticks.

Dinner: Shrimp-and-steak kabobs (made with shrimp, steak cubes, green pepper, onion and tomato). ⅓ cup *brown rice* with butter. Steamed broccoli with butter. Mixed-greens salad tossed with sesame-oil-and-lime-juice dressing.

Day 12

Breakfast: Soy sausage, mushroom and tofu scramble. ½ *grapefruit*.

Snack: Liver paté. Carrot sticks. Small handful *grapes*.

Lunch: Chicken fajitas (made with grilled chicken, bell peppers, tomato, cilantro, onion and sour cream) 1 *corn tortilla*.

Snack: Pickled herring and sour cream. 2 low-carbohydrate *whole-grain crackers*.

Dinner: Pot roast. ⅓ cup mashed *potatoes* with butter. Collard greens with butter. Mixed-greens salad with crumbled Gorgonzola cheese, ¼ sliced *pear* and drizzled with olive-oil-and-vinegar dressing.

Day 13

Breakfast: Chicken and mozzarella-cheese omelet. ⅓ cup *oatmeal* with butter and cream. 3 ounces *vegetable juice*.

Snack: ½ serving *Tofu "Egg" Salad* (see recipe, page 330). Carrot sticks.

Lunch: Steak salad (made with strips of steak, on a bed of salad greens, cucumber and tomato tossed with olive-oil-and-vinegar dressing). 1 cup cubed *honeydew melon*.

Snack: ⅓ cup *hummus*. Carrot and celery sticks.

Dinner: Broiled fish. ⅓ cup brown *rice*. Roasted eggplant. Spinach salad tossed with olive-oil-and-vinegar dressing.

Day 14

Breakfast: Eggs over-easy. Nitrate-free bacon. 1 slice buttered low-carbohydrate *toast*. 3 ounces *vegetable juice*.

Snack: Swiss cheese. Small handful *grapes*.

Lunch: *Cottage Cheese Salad with Chopped Vegetables* (see recipe, page 328). ½ small *apple*.

Snack: Nitrate-free sausage wrapped in one small *corn tortilla*.

Dinner: Roast leg of lamb. ⅓ cup *couscous* with butter. Zucchini with butter. Cucumber salad with minced fresh dill mixed with sour-cream-and-vinegar dressing.

Day 15

Breakfast: Spinach, mushroom and Brie-cheese omelet. ¼ cup roasted *potatoes*.

Snack: ¼ cup *sunflower seeds*.

Lunch: *Cashew* chicken salad (made with diced chicken and ⅛ cup *cashews*) on a bed of salad greens tossed with olive-oil-and-vinegar dressing. ¼ cup fresh cubed *pineapple*.

Snack: String cheese. 1 *apricot*.

Dinner: Classic Beef Stroganoff (see recipe, page 333). ⅓ cup *brown rice*. Steamed asparagus with butter. Mixed-greens salad tossed with olive-oil-and-vinegar dressing.

Day 16

Breakfast: Nitrate-free sausages. ½ cup *grits* with butter and cream. Tomato slices.

Snack: 1 tablespoon *peanut butter* with ¼ small banana.

Lunch: Deviled eggs on a bed of greens with ½ cup *beets*, green peppers and tomatoes tossed with olive-oil-and-vinegar dressing. ¾ cup fresh sliced *strawberries*.

Snack: ⅓ cup *hummus*. Carrot, bell pepper and celery sticks.

Dinner: Lamb chops. String beans with butter. Mixed-greens salad tossed with olive-oil-and-vinegar dressing. ½ cup unsweetened *applesauce*.

Day 17

Breakfast: 2 scrambled eggs. ½ cup *cottage cheese.* ½ *grapefruit.*

Snack: Turkey and Swiss cheese. 1 tablespoon *raisins.*

Lunch: Hamburger (made with 2 patties, lettuce, onion, tomato, mayonnaise on 1 slice low-carbohydrate *bread*). ½ medium fresh-sliced *peach* with unsweetened whipped cream.

Snack: String cheese. ¼ cup *pistachio* nuts.

Dinner: Liver and onions. ½ cup peas with butter. Cucumber salad mixed with sour-cream-and-vinegar dressing.

Day 18

Breakfast: Scrambled eggs with onions and bell peppers. Nitrate-free sausages. 1 slice buttered *whole-grain toast* or 2 slices buttered low-carbohydrate *toast.*

Snack: One cup *cottage cheese.* Carrot sticks.

Lunch: Beefsteak tomato stuffed with tuna salad (made with tuna, minced onions, celery and mayonnaise topped with ½ sliced *avocado.*)

Snack: ¼ cup *walnuts.* ½ small *apple.*

Dinner: Meat loaf (made without breadcrumbs). ½ cup *potato salad* (made with potatoes, hard-boiled egg, celery, onion, mayonnaise and mustard). Mushrooms and green beans with butter.

Day 19

Breakfast: Hard-boiled eggs. ⅓ cup *oatmeal* with butter and cream. ½ medium *orange*.

Snack: 2 tablespoons *peanut butter* on celery.

Lunch: Chicken taco (made with chicken, tomato, lettuce, sour cream and salsa). 1 *corn tortilla*.

Snack: Mozzarella cheese. ½ cup *cherries*.

Dinner: Grilled salmon with butter and lemon. ½ cup *polenta*. Cauliflower with butter and Parmesan cheese. Mixed-greens salad with tomato, cucumber and olives, tossed with olive-oil-and-vinegar dressing.

Day 20

Breakfast: ½ serving *Tofu "Egg" Salad* (see recipe, page 330). ¾ cup strawberries with unsweetened whipping cream.

Snack: ¼ cup *pumpkin seeds*.

Lunch: Cheeseburger (made with hamburger patty, mozzarella cheese, lettuce, tomato, onion and mayonnaise) on two slices low-carbohydrate *bread*.

Snack: Liver paté. 2 low-carbohydrate *whole-grain crackers*.

Dinner: Broccoli Cheese Pie (see recipe, page 332). Mixed-greens salad tossed with olive-oil-and-vinegar dressing. ½ cup *raspberries* with unsweetened whipping cream.

Day 21

Breakfast: Steak and eggs. ¼ cup sautéed *potatoes* with onions and mushrooms. 3 ounces *vegetable juice.*

Snack: Feta cheese on 2 low-carbohydrate *whole-grain crackers.*

Lunch: Salmon salad (made with salmon, onions, capers, celery and mayonnaise). ½ sliced *avocado* and sliced tomato.

Snack: ¼ cup cashews.

Dinner: Grilled *tofu.* 1 cup steamed *carrots* with butter. Mixed-greens salad tossed with olive-oil-and-vinegar dressing.

Day 22

Breakfast: Goat cheese and mushroom omelet. Nitrate-free sausages. 1 slice buttered *whole-grain toast,* or 2 slices buttered low-carbohydrate *toast.* Sliced tomatoes.

Snack: Swiss cheese. Small handful *grapes.*

Lunch: Tuna salad (made with tuna, diced celery and mayonnaise), on a bed of greens tossed with olive-oil-and-vinegar dressing and topped with sliced ½ *avocado.*

Snack: ½ cup cottage cheese. ¼ cup unsweetened *applesauce.*

Dinner: Roast chicken. ⅓ cup *couscous* with butter. Mixed vegetables with butter. Mixed-greens salad with cucumber slices and tomato wedges, tossed with olive-oil-and-vinegar dressing.

Day 23

Breakfast: Scrambled eggs with cream cheese. 1 slice buttered *whole-grain toast,* or 2 slices buttered low-carbohydrate *toast.* Sliced tomatoes.

Snack: Camembert cheese. ¾ cup *strawberries* with unsweetened whipping cream.

Lunch: Grilled chicken breast and spinach salad (made with spinach greens, tomatoes, mushrooms and two small mandarin *oranges* tossed with olive-oil-and-vinegar dressing and topped with grilled chicken breasts).

Snack: ⅓ cup *hummus.* Carrot and celery sticks.

Dinner: Eggplant Parmigiana (see recipe, page 334). Mixed-greens salad with cucumber slices and tomato wedges, tossed with olive-oil-and-vinegar dressing.

Day 24

Breakfast: 2 hard-boiled eggs. 2 tablespoons *almond butter* on ½ small *apple.*

Snack: Roast beef and Swiss cheese. 2 low-carbohydrate *whole-grain crackers.*

Lunch: Turkey cheeseburger (made with turkey patty, mozzarella cheese, lettuce, tomato, onion and mayonnaise) on two slices low-carbohydrate *bread.*

Snack: 2 tablespoons *peanut butter* on celery sticks.

Dinner: Stir fry (made with sautéed chicken and/or tofu, garlic, basil, red bell peppers, mushrooms) over ⅓ cup *brown rice.* Sliced tomato, buffalo mozzarella cheese, fresh basil leaves drizzled with olive-oil-and-vinegar dressing.

Day 25

Breakfast: Shrimp omelet (made with shrimp and scallions). 6 ounces *tomato juice*.

Snack: One cup *cottage cheese*. Carrot sticks.

Lunch: Chicken Caesar salad (made with romaine lettuce, grilled chicken, anchovies and Parmesan cheese tossed with olive-oil-and-lemon dressing). 1 cup *cherries*.

Snack: Liver paté on 2 low-carbohydrate *whole-grain crackers*.

Dinner: New York steak. ½ baked potato with butter, sour cream and chives. Steamed broccoli and butter. Mixed-greens salad with olive-oil-and-vinegar dressing.

Day 26

Breakfast: Breakfast sandwich (made with scrambled eggs, nitrate-free ham, Muenster cheese, and sliced tomato) on 2 slices buttered low-carbohydrate *toast*.

Snack: ½ cup *cottage cheese*. ¼ cup fresh cubed *melon*.

Lunch: Curried chicken salad (made with diced chicken breast, celery, onion, 1 small, cubed *apple*, and mayonnaise and curry powder to taste). Sprinkling of *sunflower seeds*.

Snack: Sardines. 2 low-carbohydrate *whole-grain crackers*.

Dinner: Roast chicken. 1 *artichoke* with melted butter. Mixed-greens salad with tomatoes, onions, cucumber and sprouts. Tossed with olive-oil-and-vinegar dressing.

Day 27

Breakfast: Nitrate-free sausages. ½ cup *grits* with butter and unsweetened cream. Sliced tomatoes.

Snack: Deviled eggs. ½ medium *orange*.

Lunch: Tuna melt on 2 slices buttered low-carbohydrate *toast* with mozzarella cheese. Mixed-greens salad with tomatoes, onions, cucumber and sprouts tossed with olive-oil-and-lemon-juice dressing.

Snack: 2 tablespoons *almond butter* on celery sticks.

Dinner: Roast pork loin. Mixed vegetables with butter. 1/3 cup *lentils* with butter. Mixed-greens salad with tomatoes, onions, cucumber and sprouts, tossed with olive-oil-and-vinegar dressing.

Day 28

Breakfast: Eggs over-easy. Nitrate-free bacon. 1 slice buttered low-carbohydrate *toast*. 6 ounces *carrot juice*.

Snack: Mozzarella cheese with ½ small *apple*.

Lunch: Nitrate-free Polish sausages and sauerkraut. ½ cup boiled *potatoes* with butter.

Snack: ¼ cup *sunflower seeds*.

Dinner: Broiled swordfish. 1 medium *corn* on the cob with butter. Coleslaw (made with shredded cabbage, carrots and onions with mayonnaise-and-vinegar dressing).

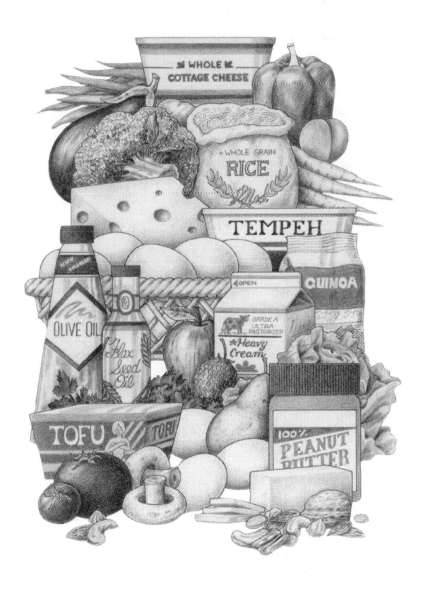

**Figure 27-3. What a Vegetarian's Groceries Look Like
on the Schwarzbein Program**

Four Weeks of Healing Program Vegetarian Meal Plans

Day 1

Breakfast: Scrambled eggs with soy sausages. ⅔ cup *oatmeal* with butter and cream. Sliced tomatoes.

Snack: Muenster cheese. ¼ cup *sunflower seeds*.

Lunch: *Tofu "Egg" Salad* (see recipe, page 330) in beefsteak tomato. Carrot sticks.

Snack: ¼ cup *almonds*. String cheese.

Dinner: Stir-fry tofu with snow peas, mushrooms, scallions and sprinkling of *peanuts*. ⅓ cup *brown rice*. Spinach salad with olive-oil-and-vinegar dressing.

Day 2

Breakfast: Annette Matrisciano's Cheesy Eggs (see recipe, page 322). 1 slice buttered low-carbohydrate *toast*. 3 ounces *vegetable juice*.

Snack: 2 tablespoons *peanut butter* on celery sticks.

Lunch: Grilled *tofu*. Coleslaw (made with shredded cabbage, carrots and onions with mayonnaise-and-vinegar dressing).

Snack: ⅓ cup *hummus* with carrot, bell pepper and celery sticks.

Dinner: *Eggplant Parmigiana* (see recipe, page 334). ⅓ cup *brown rice* with butter. Mixed-greens salad tossed with olive-oil-and-vinegar dressing.

Day 3

Breakfast: Spinach and feta-cheese omelet. 1 cup cubed *honeydew melon.*

Snack: Swiss cheese. 1 tablespoon *raisins.*

Lunch: Grilled tofu Caesar salad (made with grilled tofu, romaine lettuce and Parmesan cheese tossed with olive-oil-and-lemon dressing). 1 medium *orange.*

Snack: 1½ tablespoons *cashew butter* on celery sticks.

Dinner: *Tempeh* burger with sautéed mushrooms. ½ cup oven-roasted *potatoes.* Steamed zucchini with butter. Carrot salad with mayonnaise-and-vinegar dressing.

Day 4

Breakfast: Scrambled eggs. Sliced tomatoes. ⅔ cup *oatmeal* with butter and cream.

Snack: Mozzarella cheese. 2 low-carbohydrate *whole-grain crackers.*

Lunch: Mixed-greens salad with tofu, sun-dried tomatoes, Greek olives, ¼ cup *walnuts* tossed with olive-oil-and-vinegar dressing. ¾ cup fresh cubed *pineapple.*

Snack: 1 cup *cottage cheese.* Carrot sticks.

Dinner: *Tempeh* and Monterey Jack or Gruyère cheese "quesadilla" with 1 *corn tortilla,* topped with salsa and sour cream. Mixed-greens salad of greens, tomatoes and jicama tossed with olive-oil-and-lime juice dressing.

Day 5

Breakfast: Scrambled eggs with mushrooms and spinach. ⅔ cup *oatmeal* with butter and cream.

Snack: String cheese. ½ small *apple*.

Lunch: Grilled tofu dogs, on ½ whole-grain bun with mustard and mayonnaise. Carrot and celery sticks.

Snack: Deviled eggs. ½ medium *orange*.

Dinner: Nancy Deville's Crustless Spinach and Mushroom Quiche (see recipe, page 323). Mixed-greens salad with tomatoes and tossed with olive-oil-and-vinegar dressing and topped with ½ sliced *avocado*.

Day 6

Breakfast: Soy sausages. 2 eggs over-easy. 2 slices buttered low-carbohydrate *toast*. Sliced tomatoes.

Snack: Swiss cheese. 1 *fig*.

Lunch: Anytime Soup (see recipe, page 331). 2 low carbohydrate *whole-grain crackers*.

Snack: 2 tablespoons almond butter on 2 low-carbohydrate *whole-grain crackers*.

Dinner: Tofu, mushroom, bell pepper kabobs. ⅓ cup *black bean* chili topped with sour cream and grated mozzarella cheese. Mixed-greens salad with tomatoes and tossed with olive-oil-and-vinegar dressing.

Day 7

Breakfast: San Francisco Joe's Special (see recipe, page 324, substitute crumbled soy sausage for meat). 1 medium *orange*.

Snack: ½ cup *cottage cheese*. ¼ cup unsweetened *applesauce*.

Lunch: Grilled Monterey Jack or Gruyère cheese and tomato sandwich on 2 slices low-carbohydrate *bread*. Carrot sticks.

Snack: Swiss cheese. ¼ cup *cashews*.

Dinner: Grilled *tofu*. ⅓ cup *kasha*. Steamed broccoli with butter and Parmesan cheese. Mixed-greens salad tossed with olive-oil-and-vinegar dressing.

Day 8

Breakfast: Spinach and mushroom omelet. 1 cup cubed *cantaloupe*.

Snack: ½ serving *Tofu "Egg" Salad* (see recipe, page 330). Carrot sticks.

Lunch: Chef's salad (made with Swiss cheese, hard-boiled eggs, salad greens and tomatoes), tossed with olive-oil-and-vinegar dressing. ½ buttered *whole-grain roll*.

Snack: ⅓ cup *hummus* with carrot and celery sticks.

Dinner: Barbecued *tofu* (do not use sweetened or bottled barbecue sauce). ½ *baked potato* with butter, sour cream and chives. Mixed-greens salad tossed with olive-oil-and-vinegar dressing.

Day 9

Breakfast: Scrambled eggs with mushrooms and cream cheese. ½ cup sautéed *potatoes*. Tomato slices.

Snack: String cheese. ¾ cup sliced *strawberries* with unsweetened whipping cream.

Lunch: *Tofu "Egg" salad* (see recipe, page 330). Carrot sticks. Sliced tomatoes.

Snack: Swiss cheese. ¼ cup *almonds*.

Dinner: Greek-Style Baked Fish (see recipe, page 335, and substitute drained and pressed tofu for fish). ⅓ cup *brown rice* with butter. Mixed-greens salad tossed with olive-oil-and-vinegar dressing.

Day 10

Breakfast: Scrambled eggs with soy sausages, onions and bell pepper. 1 slice buttered *whole-grain toast*, or 2 slices buttered low-carbohydrate *toast*.

Snack: 4 tablespoons *almond butter* on celery sticks.

Lunch: Grilled *tempeh* and spinach salad with ¼ cup diced jicama and bean sprouts tossed with sesame-oil-and-lime-juice dressing.

Snack: Mozzarella cheese. ½ cup *cherries*.

Dinner: Stir-fry tofu with snow peas and mushrooms. ⅓ cup *brown rice*. Mixed-greens salad with water chestnuts and bean sprouts, tossed with olive-oil-and-vinegar dressing.

Day 11

Breakfast: Sun-dried tomato and goat cheese tofu scramble. 1 slice buttered *whole-grain toast*, or 2 slices buttered low-carbohydrate *toast*. 3 ounces *vegetable juice*.

Snack: Buffalo mozzarella cheese on 2 low-carbohydrate *whole-grain crackers*.

Lunch: Tofu hot dogs on ½ *whole-grain bun* with mayonnaise and mustard. Coleslaw (made with shredded cabbage, carrots and onions with mayonnaise-and-vinegar dressing).

Snack: ⅓ cup *hummus* on celery sticks.

Dinner: Tofu kabobs (made with tofu, green pepper, onion and mushrooms). ⅓ cup *brown rice* with butter. Steamed broccoli with butter. Mixed-greens salad tossed with olive-oil-and-vinegar dressing.

Day 12

Breakfast: Soy sausage, mushroom and tofu scramble. ½ *grapefruit*.

Snack: Hard-boiled egg. Vegetable paté on 2 low-carbohydrate *whole-grain crackers*.

Lunch: Tofu fajitas (made with grilled tofu, bell peppers, tomato, cilantro, onion and sour cream) 1 *corn tortilla*.

Snack: Swiss cheese. ½ small *apple*.

Dinner: Baked ricotta-cheese stuffed bell peppers (made with ricotta cheese, egg, Parmesan cheese, onions and garlic). ⅓ cup *couscous*. Mixed-greens salad tossed with olive-oil-and-vinegar dressing.

Day 13

Breakfast: Scrambled tofu with zucchini and mushrooms. 1 small *apple*.

Snack: ½ serving *Tofu "Egg" Salad* (see recipe, page 330). Celery sticks.

Lunch: Grilled *tempeh* salad (made with grilled strips of *tempeh*, on a bed of salad greens, cucumber and tomato tossed with olive-oil-and-vinegar dressing).

Snack: ⅓ cup *hummus*. Carrot and celery sticks.

Dinner: *Eggplant Parmigiana* (see recipe, page 334). ⅓ cup *brown rice*. Spinach salad tossed with olive-oil-and-vinegar dressing.

Day 14

Breakfast: Soy sausage and eggs over-easy. 1 slice buttered *whole-grain toast*, or 2 slices buttered low-carbohydrate *toast*. Sliced tomatoes.

Snack: String cheese. 1 *apricot*.

Lunch: Greek salad (made with grilled tofu, Kalamata olives, feta cheese and tomatoes on a bed of spinach tossed with olive-oil-and-lemon-juice dressing). Small handful *grapes*.

Snack: Camembert cheese. 1 cup *raspberries* with unsweetened whipping cream.

Dinner: Tofu Stroganoff (see Classic Beef Stroganoff recipe, page 333, substitute tofu for meat and vegetable broth for meat broth). ⅓ cup *brown rice*. Steamed asparagus with butter. Mixed-greens salad tossed with olive-oil-and-vinegar dressing.

Day 15

Breakfast: Spinach, mushroom and Brie omelet. ¼ cup roasted *potatoes*.

Snack: Swiss cheese. Small handful *grapes*.

Lunch: *Cottage Cheese Salad with Chopped Vegetables* (see recipe, page 328). 1 small *apple*.

Snack: Soy sausage wrapped in one *corn tortilla*.

Dinner: Baked tofu with mozzarella cheese. ⅓ cup *couscous* with butter. Zucchini with butter. Cucumber salad mixed with sour-cream-and-vinegar dressing.

Day 16

Breakfast: Soy sausages. ½ cup *grits* with butter and cream. Tomato slices.

Snack: 1 tablespoon *peanut butter* with ¼ small *banana*.

Lunch: Deviled eggs on a bed of greens with ½ cup *beets*, green peppers and tomatoes tossed with olive-oil-and-vinegar dressing. ¾ cup fresh sliced *strawberries*.

Snack: ⅓ cup *hummus*. Carrot, bell pepper and celery sticks.

Dinner: Grilled *tempeh*. ½ cup unsweetened *applesauce*. String beans with butter. Mixed-greens salad tossed with olive-oil-and-vinegar dressing.

Day 17

Breakfast: Hard-boiled eggs. 1 cup *cottage cheese*. ½ *grapefruit*.

Snack: Swiss cheese. 1 tablespoon *raisins*.

Lunch: Tofu burger (made with 2 tofu patties, lettuce, onion, tomato and mayonnaise on 1 slice low-carbohydrate *bread*). ½ medium fresh sliced *peach* with unsweetened whipping cream.

Snack: ¼ cup *pistachio nuts*. String cheese.

Dinner: Sun-dried tomato and goat-cheese omelet. Sautéed mushrooms. ⅓ cup roasted *potatoes*. Mixed-greens salad with sprouts, tossed with olive-oil-and-vinegar dressing.

Day 18

Breakfast: Scrambled eggs with onions and bell peppers. Soy sausages. 1 slice buttered *whole-grain toast* or 2 slices buttered low-carbohydrate *toast*.

Snack: ½ cup *cottage cheese*. Carrot sticks.

Lunch: Beefsteak tomato stuffed with ½ serving *Tofu "Egg" Salad* (see recipe, page 330). 2 low-carbohydrate *whole-grain crackers*.

Snack: ½ small *apple*. String cheese.

Dinner: Stir-fry tofu with broccoli, scallions and sprinkling *almonds*. ⅓ cup brown *rice*. Spinach salad with mushrooms and bean sprouts tossed with sesame-oil-and-lime-juice dressing.

Day 19

Breakfast: Spicy tofu frittata (see Spicy Chicken Frittata recipe, page 326, substitute tofu for chicken). ½ cup *grits* with butter and cream.

Snack: 2 tablespoons *peanut butter* on celery.

Lunch: Tofu burger topped with mozzarella cheese and sautéed mushrooms. ½ cup *potato salad* (made with *potatoes*, hard-boiled egg, celery, onion, mayonnaise and mustard).

Snack: Mozzarella cheese. ½ cup *cherries*.

Dinner: Grilled *tempeh*. ½ cup *polenta*. Cauliflower with butter and Parmesan cheese. Mixed-greens salad with tomato, cucumber and olives tossed with olive-oil-and-vinegar dressing.

Day 20

Breakfast: *Tofu "Egg" salad* (see recipe, page 330). ½ whole-grain buttered, *English muffin*. Sliced tomatoes.

Snack: Swiss cheese. ¼ cup *pumpkin seeds*.

Lunch: *Tempeh* burger (made with *tempeh* patties, mozzarella cheese, lettuce, tomato, onion and mayonnaise) on two slices low-carbohydrate *bread*.

Snack: Hard-boiled eggs. Vegetable paté. 2 low-carbohydrate *whole-grain crackers*.

Dinner: Broccoli Cheese Pie (see recipe, page 332). Mixed-greens salad tossed with olive-oil-and-vinegar dressing. ½ cup *raspberries* with unsweetened whipping cream.

Day 21

Breakfast: Spinach and Brie-cheese omelet with soy bacon. ¼ cup roasted *potatoes*.

Snack: 1 tablespoon *almond butter* on 2 low-carbohydrate *whole-grain crackers*.

Lunch: *Cottage Cheese* Salad with Chopped Vegetables (see recipe, page 328). ½ small *apple*.

Snack: Provolone cheese. ¼ cup *cashews*.

Dinner: Tofu meatballs (made with tofu, egg, sautéed onions and garlic and Parmesan cheese). ⅓ cup mashed *potatoes*. Steamed broccoli with butter. Mixed-greens salad with crumbled bleu cheese tossed with olive-oil-and-vinegar dressing.

Day 22

Breakfast: Soy sausages. ½ cup *oatmeal* with butter and cream.

Snack: Swiss cheese. Small handful *grapes*.

Lunch: Grilled tofu tostada (made with grilled tofu, grated mozzarella cheese, lettuce, sour cream and salsa mounded on 1 *corn tortilla*).

Snack: ½ cup *cottage cheese*. ¼ cup unsweetened *applesauce*.

Dinner: Goat cheese, sun-dried tomato and mushroom omelet. Mixed-greens salad with tomatoes, cucumber and bell pepper tossed with olive-oil-and-vinegar dressing. ¾ cup *blueberries* with unsweetened whipping cream.

Day 23

Breakfast: Scrambled eggs with cream cheese. 1 slice buttered *whole-grain toast*, or 2 slices buttered low-carbohydrate *toast*. Sliced tomatoes.

Snack: Camembert cheese. ¾ cup *strawberries* with unsweetened whipped cream.

Lunch: Grilled tofu and spinach salad (made with spinach greens, tomatoes, mushrooms and two small mandarin *oranges* tossed with olive-oil-and-vinegar dressing and topped with grilled tofu).

Snack: ⅓ cup *hummus*. Carrot and celery sticks.

Dinner: Eggplant Parmigiana (see recipe, page 334). Mixed-greens salad with cucumber slices and tomato wedges tossed with olive-oil-and-vinegar dressing.

Day 24

Breakfast: 2 hard-boiled eggs. 2 tablespoons *almond butter* on ½ small *apple*.

Snack: Mozzarella cheese. 2 low-carbohydrate *whole-grain crackers*.

Lunch: Pita pocket (made with grated mozzarella cheese, mushrooms, tomato, shredded lettuce, sprouts in 1 small *whole-grain pita* bread). Carrot and celery sticks.

Snack: 2 tablespoons *peanut butter* on celery sticks.

Dinner: Stir fry (made with sautéed tofu, garlic, basil, red bell peppers and mushrooms) over ⅓ cup *brown rice*. Spinach, bean sprout, jicama, bell pepper salad tossed with sesame-oil-and-lime-juice dressing.

Day 25

Breakfast: Poached eggs with 2 slices buttered low-carbohydrate *toast*. Sliced tomatoes.

Snack: One cup *cottage cheese*. Carrot sticks.

Lunch: Grilled tofu Caesar salad (made with grilled tofu, romaine lettuce and Parmesan cheese tossed with olive-oil-and-lemon dressing). 1 cup *cherries*.

Snack: Hard-boiled egg. Mushroom paté on 2 low-carbohydrate *whole-grain crackers*.

Dinner: Grilled *tempeh* with sautéed scallions and mushrooms. ⅓ cup *millet*. Steamed asparagus with butter. Coleslaw (made with shredded cabbage, carrots and onions with mayonnaise-and-vinegar dressing).

Day 26

Breakfast: Breakfast sandwich (made with scrambled eggs, soy bacon, Muenster cheese, sliced tomato) on 2 slices buttered low-carbohydrate *toast*.

Snack: ½ cup *cottage cheese*. ¼ cup fresh cubed *melon*.

Lunch: Curried tofu salad (made with diced tofu, celery, onion, 1 small, cubed *apple*, mayonnaise and curry powder to taste) with sprinkling of *sunflower seeds*.

Snack: Mozzarella cheese. 2 low-carbohydrate *whole-grain crackers*.

Dinner: *Chinese tofu salad* (See Chinese Chicken Salad recipe, page 327, substitute tofu for chicken).

San Francisco Joe's Special
(scrambled eggs, hamburger meat and spinach)

Makes 2 servings • Each serving: 49 grams protein • trace carbohydrate

1 bunch spinach equal to about 1 cup cooked spinach, well-drained and chopped; or 8-ounce package frozen spinach, thawed, drained and chopped

½ pound lean hamburger meat

2 tablespoons unsalted butter

½ cup chopped onion

1 minced garlic clove

½ teaspoon oregano

freshly ground pepper, to taste

4 eggs

2 tablespoons grated Parmesan cheese

Wash spinach well, removing stems. With water still clinging to leaves, place in a heavy medium saucepan with a tight-fitting lid. Turn heat to medium-high and steam until leaves are wilted, about 2 to 3 minutes. Drain in a colander, pressing out all liquid with the back of a wooden spoon. Chop coarsely and set aside.

In a medium skillet, cook hamburger over medium heat until browned, breaking apart lumps with a wooden spoon. Remove meat from pan, drain fat and set aside.

In a large nonstick skillet, melt butter over a medium-high heat. When butter is hot and bubbly, add onion and garlic and sauté until softened, about 5 minutes. Stir in oregano and black pepper. Add spinach and hamburger meat and stir until spinach is heated through.

In a small bowl, using a fork, beat eggs and pour over meat mixture. Gently stir egg/meat mixture with a wooden spoon until cooked to your liking. Sprinkle with Parmesan cheese. Taste, and adjust seasonings. Serve immediately.

Day 27

Breakfast: Soy sausages. ½ cup *grits* with butter and whipping cream. Sliced tomatoes.

Snack: Deviled eggs. ½ medium *orange*.

Lunch: Tofu melt (made with grilled tofu and grated Muenster cheese on 2 slices buttered low-carbohydrate *bread*). Mixed-greens salad with tomatoes, onions, cucumber and sprouts tossed with olive-oil-and-vinegar dressing.

Snack: 2 tablespoons *almond butter* on celery sticks.

Dinner: Baked *tempeh*. ⅓ cup lentils with butter. Mixed vegetables with butter. Mixed-greens salad with tomatoes, onions, cucumber and sprouts tossed with olive-oil-and-vinegar dressing.

Day 28

Breakfast: Three-minute eggs with soy bacon. 1 slice buttered *whole-grain toast*, or 2 slices buttered low-carbohydrate *toast*.

Snack: Mozzarella cheese with ½ small *apple*.

Lunch: Spicy tofu sausages and sauerkraut. ½ cup boiled *potatoes* with butter.

Snack: Swiss cheese. ¼ cup *sunflower seeds*.

Dinner: Broiled *tempeh*. 1 medium corn on the cob with butter. Coleslaw (made with shredded cabbage, carrots and onions with mayonnaise-and-vinegar dressing).

Breakfast Entrées

Annette Matrisciano's Cheesy Eggs

Makes 2 servings. Each serving: 25 grams protein • 3 grams carbohydrate

4 eggs

3 ounces cream cheese, cut into
   ½-inch cubes

¼ cup grated Parmesan cheese

freshly ground black pepper,
   to taste

2 tablespoons unsalted butter

1 minced garlic clove

In a small bowl, beat eggs with cream-cheese cubes, Parmesan cheese and black pepper. Set aside.

In a medium nonstick skillet, melt butter over medium-high heat. When butter is hot and bubbly, add garlic and sauté about half a minute. Pour egg mixture into skillet. Stir and fold gently until cream cheese is melted and eggs are cooked to your liking. Serve immediately.

Nancy Deville's Crustless Spinach and Mushroom Quiche

Makes 8 servings. Each serving: 14 grams protein • trace carbohydrate

2 bunches spinach equal to about
   2 cups cooked spinach, well-
   drained and chopped; or
   16-ounces package frozen
   spinach, thawed, drained and
   chopped

6 tablespoons unsalted butter

1 medium chopped red onion

2 cups chopped white
   mushrooms

6 eggs

2 cups all-dairy heavy cream

freshly ground black pepper, to
taste

2 cups each grated Monterey Jack
and Gruyère cheese

Wash spinach well, removing stems. Put in a microwaveable container with one inch of water and microwave for about 2 to 3 minutes, or until spinach is wilted. Drain in a colander. Squeeze all water from spinach until it feels "dry." Chop fine and set aside.

Preheat oven to 350°. In a medium nonstick skillet, melt butter over medium-low heat. When butter is hot and bubbly, add onion and mushrooms and sauté until soft and all liquid from the mushrooms has cooked away, about 10 minutes.

In the meantime, in a medium bowl, using a fork, whisk eggs, cream and black pepper until well blended. Add grated cheese and spinach and mix well. Slowly add mushroom and onion mixture to egg mixture and mix well.

Butter a 9 x 13-inch baking pan. Pour in custard mixture. Bake 35 to 45 minutes until custard is set and knife comes out clean. Do not overcook.

Soy Sausage Tofu Scramble

Makes 2 servings • Each serving: 54 grams protein • 12 grams carbohydrate

2 tablespoons pure-pressed extra
  virgin olive oil

4 diced soy sausages

1 pound firm tofu, drained,
  pressed and crumbled

freshly ground black papper,
  to taste

1 teaspoon dried thyme

½ cup grated mozzarella cheese

In a 10-inch nonstick skillet, heat oil over medium-high heat. When oil is hot, add soy sausages and sauté until browned. Add tofu, black pepper and thyme, and sauté until heated through, gently stirring tofu mixture with a wooden spoon. Add mozzarella cheese and cook until melted. Serve hot.

Spicy Chicken Frittata

Makes 2 servings • Each serving: 30 grams protein • trace carbohydrate

1 chicken breast

2 bay leaves

4 eggs

*2 tablespoons all-dairy
  heavy cream*

*freshly ground black pepper,
  to taste*

dash cayenne pepper

Filling

2 tablespoons unsalted butter

½ cup diced red bell pepper

¼ cup diced red onion

1 teaspoon ground cumin

1 teaspoon oregano

1 cup diced green olives

2 tablespoons unsalted butter

*1 tablespoon grated
  Parmesan cheese*

*2 teaspoons finely chopped fresh
  parsley,* or *cilantro, for garnish*

In a medium covered skillet, poach chicken with 2 bay leaves in 1 inch of water over medium heat until cooked through, about 20 minutes. *Do not overcook.* Let cool and shred with your fingers.

Preheat broiler. In a medium bowl, using a fork, whisk eggs, cream, black pepper and cayenne pepper. Set aside.

In a 10-inch flameproof skillet, melt 2 tablespoons butter over medium-high heat. When butter is hot and bubbly, add bell peppers and onion and sauté until softened, about 5 minutes. Add cumin, oregano, olives and shredded chicken, and cook 2 minutes, stirring occasionally. Remove from pan and set aside.

In the same skillet, melt remaining 2 tablespoons butter over medium-high heat. When butter is hot and bubbly, add egg mixture. As eggs cook, lift edges to allow uncooked egg to seep underneath. When bottom is set but top is till moist, spread chicken filling over egg and place under broiler. Broil 1 to 2 minutes, checking frequently, until top is golden and puffed up. Sprinkle with Parmesan cheese. Garnish plates with finely chopped parsley (or cilantro). Serve hot or at room temperature.

Salads and Soups

Chinese Chicken Salad

Makes 4 main-course servings • Each serving: 33 grams protein • 3 grams carbohydrate

2 cups cooked julienned chicken

1 medium jicama, peeled and
sliced into matchstick pieces; or
12 sliced water chestnuts,
rinsed and drained

6 cups mixed salad greens

½ cup dry roasted peanuts

1 tablespoon minced fresh
cilantro

3 celery stalks, sliced into thin
sticks, then cut diagonally into
1½" pieces

3 minced scallions

1 red bell pepper, cut into
very thin strips

Chinese Chicken Salad Dressing

In a large bowl, combine chicken, jicama or water chestnuts, celery, scallions and bell pepper. Mix well.

Line 4 individual plates with washed and dried salad greens. Arrange chicken and vegetables over greens. Sprinkle peanuts and minced cilantro over the top. Spoon Chinese Chicken Salad Dressing over the salad. Serve remaining dressing on the side.

Chinese Chicken Salad Dressing

1 teaspoon grated fresh
ginger root

2 minced garlic cloves

1 tablespoon low-sodium
tamari soy sauce

2 tablespoons fresh lime juice

¼ cup pure-pressed sesame oil

½ cup pure-pressed mayonnaise

In a blender or food processor, blend all ingredients until smooth, or place ingredients in a jar with a tight-fitting lid and shake vigorously until well blended. Taste, and adjust seasonings.

Cottage Cheese Salad with Chopped Vegetables

Makes 2 servings • Each serving: 14 grams protein • 6 grams carbohydrate

2 finely diced carrots

3 finely chopped scallions

1 finely chopped red bell pepper

3 finely chopped celery stalks

1 tablespoon minced fresh parsley

1 tablespoon minced fresh chives

2 cups cottage cheese

freshly ground black pepper, to taste

4 cups mixed salad greens

Mix all ingredients, except salad greens, with cottage cheese. Taste, and adjust seasonings. Line 4 individual plates with mixed salad greens. Mound cottage cheese salad on top. Serve immediately.

Salad Niçoise

Makes 4 servings • Each serving: 29 grams protein • 10 grams carbohydrate

16 green beans, ends trimmed

2 large red potatoes (peeled, if desired)

oil and vinegar to taste

1 head Boston or bibb lettuce, washed, with leaves torn into large pieces

2 hard-boiled eggs, sliced into quarters lengthwise

½ cup Greek, green or black olives

1 tablespoon drained and rinsed capers

13 ounces canned tuna, drained and flaked

2 medium quartered tomatoes

1 ounce canned, drained flat anchovy fillets (optional)

1 tablespoon chopped fresh basil

1 tablespoon minced scallions

Cook green beans in boiling water until just barely tender, about 5 minutes. Remove with a slotted spoon and rinse under cold water. Drain again and slice diagonally into 1-inch sections.

Cook potatoes in the same boiling water until tender, about 15 to 20 minutes. Cut into 1-inch cubes. Sprinkle potatoes with a little oil and vinegar while they are still warm. Set aside.

Line a large platter with lettuce leaves. Arrange green beans, potatoes, hard-boiled eggs, olives, capers, tuna, tomatoes and anchovies on the lettuce. Sprinkle top with chopped fresh basil and minced scallions.

Spoon oil-and-vinegar dressing to taste over salad, or serve oil and vinegar on the side. Serve immediately.

Tofu "Egg" Salad

Makes 2 servings • Each serving: 22 grams protein • 16 grams carbohydrate

1 pound firm tofu, drained, pressed and crumbled

⅓ cup mayonnaise (made from pure-pressed oil)

1 tablespoon Dijon mustard

½ cup minced celery stalks

2 teaspoons fresh lemon or lime juice

1 teaspoon dried dill

2 tablespoons minced scallions

2 tablespoons minced fresh parsley

1 tablespoon drained and rinsed capers (optional)

1½ teaspoons turmeric

freshly ground black pepper, to taste

dash cayenne pepper

In a small bowl, using a fork, mix all ingredients until well-blended. Taste, and adjust seasonings. Refrigerate 1 hour before serving.

Anytime Soup is a "prescription" soup to eat during the initial phase of "The Healing Program." If you are hungry between meals, eat Anytime soup as a snack.

Anytime Soup

Makes 8 servings • Each serving: 17 grams protein • 10 grams carbohydrate

*1 pound chicken parts or
 soup bones*

½ head shredded green cabbage

1 minced garlic clove

2 chopped celery stalks

2 pounds diced fresh tomatoes

3 chopped carrots

*2 tablespoons chopped fresh
 parsley*

*½ teaspoon dried thyme
 (optional)*

½ teapoon dried basil (optional)

*freshly ground black pepper,
 to taste*

*4 cups chicken stock or vegetable
 stock or 4 cups water*

*1-2 tablespoons fresh lemon
 juice, or 1-2 tablespoons cider
 vinegar, to taste*

In a large heavy-bottomed soup pot, bring all ingredients, except lemon juice or vinegar to a boil. Lower heat and simmer 1 hour. Remove chicken parts or soup bones. Shred chicken meat and return to pot. Add lemon juice or vinegar.

Main Entrées

Broccoli Cheese Pie

Makes 6 servings • Each serving: 16 grams protein • 6 grams carbohydrate

2 tablespoons unsalted butter

⅔ cup sliced scallions

2½ cups steamed broccoli, cut into bite-size florets, with stalks trimmed and chopped; or 20 ounces packaged frozen broccoli, thawed, drained, chopped and steamed

1½ cups whole cottage cheese or whole ricotta cheese

3 beaten eggs

2 ounces crumbled Gorgonzola or bleu cheese

¼ cup minced fresh parsley

2 tablespoons fresh slivered basil, or 2 teaspoons dried basil

3 tablespoons flour

freshly ground black pepper, to taste

dash cayenne pepper

2 tablespoons grated Parmesan cheese

Preheat oven to 350°. In a large nonstick skillet, melt butter over medium-high heat. When butter is hot and bubbly, reduce heat to medium. Add scallions and sauté until softened, about 3 minutes. In a large bowl, using a fork, blend sautéed scallions, broccoli, cottage cheese or ricotta cheese, eggs, Gorgonzola cheese, parsley, basil, flour, black pepper and cayenne pepper.

Pour filling into a buttered 9-inch baking pan or soufflé dish. Top with Parmesan cheese and bake until puffed up and golden brown, about 30 to 35 minutes. Broil for 1 minute to brown top. Let cool 5 minutes before slicing.

Classic Beef Stroganoff

Makes 4 servings • Each serving: 44 grams protein • 5 grams carbohydrate
½ cup steamed brown rice: 3 grams protein • 23 grams carbohydrate

1½ pounds beef fillet, sirloin or other boneless lean beef

freshly ground black pepper

1½ tablespoons pure-pressed monounsaturated vegetable oil

2 tablespoons unsalted butter

1 medium finely sliced onion

1 minced garlic clove

1½ tablespoons unsalted butter

1 tablespoon flour

1 cup heated beef stock (low-sodium canned)

2 teaspoons Dijon mustard

1 cup whole sour cream

1 tablespoon minced fresh parsley, for garnish

Cut beef across grain into thin diagonal strips about 1¼-inch thick. Season with pepper.

In a large, heavy skillet, heat oil over medium-high heat. When oil is hot, quickly brown meat on both sides. Remove from pan and keep warm. Drain fat from pan. Add butter and melt over medium-high heat. When butter is hot and bubbly, add onion and garlic and sauté until softened, about 5 minutes. Spoon over reserved beef.

In a large saucepan, melt butter over medium-high heat. When butter is hot and bubbly, add flour and whisk until blended. Cook 1 minute, stirring constantly. Add hot beef stock and continue whisking until well blended and thickened. Stir in mustard and sour cream, and heat until smooth and well mixed, about 3 minutes. Add meat and onion mixture and heat through. Sprinkle with minced parsley. Serve over steamed brown rice.

Eggplant Parmigiana

Makes 4 servings • Each serving: 24 grams protein • 21 grams carbohydrate

*1 large eggplant, (peeled, if
desired) cut into ½-inch slices*

¼ cup flour

*freshly ground black pepper,
to taste*

*¼ cup pure-pressed extra
virgin olive oil*

*2 cups tomato sauce
(homemade or store-bought,
no sugar added)*

1 teaspoon dried oregano

2 cups grated mozzarella cheese

½ cup grated Parmesan cheese

Preheat oven to 375°. Slice eggplant crosswise into ½-inch slices. Dredge slices with flour mixed with black pepper.

In a large nonstick skillet, heat 2 tablespoons of oil over medium-high heat. when oil is hot, add a few eggplant slices and sauté until softened and browned, about 5 minutes on each side. Repeat with remaining oil and eggplant slices.

Spread ½ cup of tomato sauce in a 9 x 13-inch baking dish. Add a single layer of eggplant slices. Top with ¾ of sauce and ½ teaspoon oregano. Sprinkle with 1 cup mozzarella cheese and ¼ cup Parmesan cheese. Make a second layer with the rest of the eggplant, tomato sauce, oregano, mozzarella cheese and Parmesan cheese. Bake, uncovered, until hot and bubbly, about 20 to 25 minutes.

Greek-Style Baked Fish

Makes 4 servings • Each serving: 51 grams protein • 3 grams carbohydrate

*four 6-ounce fish steaks
(swordfish, halibut, seabass,
salmon)*

1 red bell pepper, or ¼ cup store-bought roasted red bell pepper

*¼ cup pure-pressed extra virgin
olive oil*

2 tablespoon minced parsley

*1 tablespoon chopped fresh
oregano or 2 teaspoons dried
oregano*

grated rind of 1 lemon

¼ cup fresh lemon juice

3 minced garlic cloves

1 tablespoon Dijon mustard

*freshly ground black pepper,
to taste*

1 cup crumbled feta cheese

Preheat oven to 425°.

Rinse fish steaks under cold water and pat dry with paper towels.

If using a fresh red bell pepper, roast pepper directly over a gas flame, or under preheated broiler on a broiler rack. Using tongs, turn pepper frequently until blistered and blackened on all sides. Place pepper in a plastic bag and seal. Let steam 15 minutes. Remove from bag and peel off all charred skin. Discard skin along with seeds and dice.

Combine diced red bell pepper with remaining ingredients except for feta cheese.

Pour marinade over fish and marinate about 30 minutes, turning several times.

Arrange fish steaks in a baking dish along with marinade. Bake about 15 minutes or until fish is tender and flakes easily with a fork. Sprinkle feta cheese over top of fish, during last 5 minutes of cooking.

Some Tips for Dining Out

- At breakfast, substitute cottage cheese or sliced tomatoes for fried potatoes or hash browns.
- Do not eat the chips and bread that are brought to your table before your meal.
- Opt for a fruit-and-cheese plate for dessert.

General

Choose	Avoid
Extra vegetables instead of pasta or french fries	Alcohol, coffee, tea and sodas
	Breads and muffins
Grilled, poached, baked, roasted or broiled meats, poultry and fish	Chips
	Fried foods
	Most soups in restaurants (they contain sugar—ask for the ingredients)
Oil-and-vinegar salad dressings	
Water to drink	

Italian

Choose	Eat Less
Caesar salad with chicken or shrimp	Garlic bread sticks
Chicken marsala	Pasta
Chicken/veal piccata	
Cioppino	
Fresh mozzarella with sliced tomato	
Pesto sauce	
Seafood dishes	
1 to 2 pieces thin-crust pizza (ask to make sure there is no sugar in the tomato sauce or order sauceless pizza)	

American

Choose	Avoid
Baked/barbecued chicken (without sauce)	French fries
Broiled or grilled chicken/meat/fish	Ketchup
Burgers on half a whole-grain bun	Margarine
Grilled chicken or tuna salad[3]	Potato chips
Open-face sandwiches on whole-grain bread	
Roast turkey	
Steak	

Chinese

Request that food be prepared without MSG, sugar or soy sauce.

Choose	Eat Less
Any vegetable with meat, poultry or fish (e.g., broccoli chicken)	Chow mein
	Egg rolls
Egg-drop soup	Fried rice
Stir fries	Sweet-and-sour dishes
Tofu dishes	Wontons

French

Choose	Avoid
Bouillabaisse	Heavy cream sauces thickened
Butter sauces	with flour (ask before ordering)
Escargot	
Fish en papillote	
Poached salmon	
Roasted chicken, lamb or duck	
Salade Niçoise	
Soups	

---

[3] *Many restaurants do not use pure-pressed mayonnaise. Ask before ordering.*

Japanese

Choose	Eat Less
Boiled soybeans (as appetizer)	Noodle soups
Chicken or seafood salads	Rice noodle bowls
Grilled chicken/fish/beef dishes	Sushi
Miso soup	Tempura
Sashimi	Teriyaki sauce
Yakitori	White "sticky" rice (contains sugar)

Mexican

Choose	Avoid
Chicken/beef/seafood tostada	Fried tortilla shells
Enchiladas	Tortilla chips (unless they're made with pure-pressed oil)
Fajitas	
Grilled chicken/beef/fish dishes	
Soft tacos	

Many books on health and weight loss promise quick fixes. But if you have tried any of those approaches you understand that there is no such thing as overnight health and fitness. By reading this book you have received an education in metabolism, physiology and nutrition that you can use for the rest of your life. As you follow this program, you will achieve a level of physical and emotional health that you never thought possible. We wish you good health.

References

General Overview

Bengtsson, C., et al. "Associations of Serum Lipid Concentrations and Obesity with Mortality in Women: 20 Year Follow-up of Participants and Perspective Populations Study in Gothemberg, Sweden," *British Medical Journal* 307 (27 Nov. 1993): 1385–88.

Braunwald, Eugene, ed. *Heart Disease: A Textbook of Cardiovascular Medicine*, 5th ed. Philadelphia: W. B. Saunders, 1997.

Devlin, Thomas M., ed. *Textbook of Biochemistry*. 4th ed. New York: Wiley-Liss, 1997.

Endocrine Fellows Foundation. *Syllabus: A Review of Endocrinology: Diagnosis and Treatment*. (The Endocrinology Board Review Course). Washington, D.C.: Endocrine Fellows Foundation, October 3–7, 1993.

Greenspan, Francis S. and Peter H. Forsham, eds. *Basic and Clinical Endocrinology*. 5th ed. Los Altos, Calif.: Lange Medical Publications, 1997.

Guyton, Arthur, ed. *Textbook of Medical Physiology*. 9th ed. Philadelphia: W. B. Saunders, 1996.

Hunninghake, Donald B., ed. *The Medical Clinics of North America: Lipid Disorders*. Vol. 78. Philadelphia: W. B. Saunders, 1994.

Lehninger, Albert L., ed. *Biochemistry*. 2nd ed. New York: Worth Publishers, 1978.

Moy, C. S., ed., *Diabetes 1993 Vital Statistics.* Alexandria, Va.: American Diabetes Association, 1993.

Patton, Harry D. et al., eds. *Textbook of Physiology.* 21st ed. Vols. 1, 2. Philadelphia: W. B. Saunders,1989.

Robbins, Stanley L. and Ramzi S. Cotran, eds. *Pathologic Basis of Disease.* 2nd ed. Philadelphia: W. B. Saunders, 1979.

Scriver, Charles R., et al. *Metabolic Basis of Inherited Disease.* 6th ed. Vols. 1, 2. New York: McGraw-Hill Information Services, 1989.

Shils, Maurice E., James A. Olson, and Moshe Shike., eds. *Modern Nutrition and Health and Disease.* 8th ed. Vols. 1, 2. Philadelphia: Lea & Febiger, 1993.

U. S. Department of Health and Human Services. *National Heart, Lung and Blood Institute Fact Book.* Hyattsville, Md.: USDHHS, 1987–94.

———. *Healthy People 2000 Review 1994: National Health Promotion and Disease Prevention Objectives.* DHHS Publication No. (PHS) 95–1256–1. Hyattsville, Md.: Centers for Disease Control and Prevention, July 1995.

Wilson, Jean D., et al., eds. *Williams Textbook of Endocrinology.* 9th ed. Philadelphia: W. B. Saunders, 1998.

Wyngaarden, James B. and Lloyd H. Smith, Jr. *Cecil Textbook of Medicine.* 18th ed. Vol. 1. Philadelphia: W. B. Saunders Company, 1988.

Chapter 1

Balkau, B., et al., "Risk Factors for Early Death in Non-Insulin Dependent Diabetics and Men with Known Glucose Tolerance Status." *ACP Journal Club* 120.1 (Jan./Feb. 1994): 22.

Bassler, T. J. "Hazards of Restrictive Diets. Letters to the Editor Regarding Ischemic Deaths in Marathon Runners on a Pritikin Diet." *JAMA* 252.4 (27 July 1984): 483.

Carroll, P. B. and R. C. Eastman. "Insulin Resistance: Diagnosis and Treatment." *The Endocrinologist* 1.2 (March 1991): 89–97.

Coulston, Ann M., George C. Liu, and Gerald M. Reaven. "Plasma Glucose, Insulin and Lipid Responses to High-Carbohydrate, Low-Fat Diets in Normal Humans." *Metabolism* 32.1 (1983): 52–56.

DeFranzo, Ralph A. and Eleuterio Ferrannini. "Insulin Resistance: A Multifaceted Syndrome Responsible For NIDDM, Obesity, Hypertension, Dyslipidemia, and Atherosclerotic Cardiovascular Disease." *Diabetes Care* 14.3 (March 1991): 173–94.

Fackelmann, Kathy A. "Hidden Heart Hazards: Do High Blood Insulin Levels Foretell Heart Disease?" *Science News* 136 (16 Sept. 1989): 184–86.

Garg, Abhimanyu, Grundy, Scott M., and Roger H. Unger. "Comparison of Effects of High and Low Carbohydrate Diets on Plasma Lipoproteins and Insulin Sensitivity in Patients with Mild NIDDM." *Diabetes* 41 (19 Oct. 1992): 1278–1285.

Haffner, Steven M., et al. "Cardiovascular Risk Factors in Confirmed Prediabetic Individuals. Does the Clock for Coronary Heart Disease Start Ticking Before the Onset of Clinical Diabetes?" *JAMA* 263.21 (6 June 1990): 2893–98.

Karam, John H. "Type II Diabetes and Syndrome X: Pathogenesis and Glycemic Management." *Endocrinology and Metabolism Clinics of North America* 21.2 (June 1992): 329–50.

Kritz-Silverstein, Donna, Elizabeth Barrett-Connor, and Deborah L. Wingard. "The Effect of Parity on the Later Development of Non-Insulin-Dependent Diabetes Mellitus or Impaired Glucose Tolerance." *NEJM* 321.18 (2 Nov. 1989): 1214–19.

Moller, David E. and Jeffrey S. Flier. "Insulin Resistance-Mechanisms, Syndromes, and Implications." *NEJM* 325.13 (26 Sept. 1991): 938–48.

Pi-Sunyer, F. Xavier. "Medical Hazards of Obesity." *Annals of Internal Medicine* 119.7 (Oct. 1993): 655–59.

Reaven, Gerald M. "Syndrome X." *Blood Pressure* 1.4 (1992): 13–16.

——— . "Role of Insulin Resistance in Human Disease (Syndrome X: An Expanded Definition)." *Annual Review of Medicine* 44 (1993): 121–29.

Roses, Allen D. "Apolipoprotein E and Alzheimer's Disease." *Scientific American Science and Medicine* (Sept./Oct. 1995):16–25.

Chapter 2

Stout, Robert W. "Insulin and Atheroma: 20-Year Perspective." *Diabetes Care* 13.6 (June 1990): 631–50.

Zavaroni, Ivana, et al. "Risk Factors for Coronary Artery Disease in Healthy Persons With Hyperinsulinemia and Normal Glucose Tolerance." *NEJM* 320 (16 Mar. 1989): 702–6.

Chapter 3

Gold, Lois Swirsky, et al. "Rodent Carcinogens: Setting Priorities." *Science* 258 (Oct. 1992): 261–65.

Miller, J. C. and S. Colagiuri. "Carnivore Connection Dietary Carbohydrate and the Evolution of NIDDM." *Diabetologia* 37.12 (Dec.1994): 1280–86.

Chapter 4

Walden Health Resources. *Emotions, Overeating, and the Brain.* California: Walden Health Resources, 1993.

Chapter 5

Collier, G. R. and A. J. Sinclair. "Role of N-6 and N-3 Fatty Acids in the Dietary Treatment of Metabolic Disorders." *Annals of the New York Academy of Sciences* 683 (14 June 1993) 323–30.

Crawford, M. A., A. G. Hassam, and J. P. W. Rivers. "Essential Fatty Acid Requirement in Infancy." *American Journal of Clinical Nutrition* 31 (Dec.1978.): 2181–85.

Kern, Frank Jr., "Normal Plasma Cholesterol in an 88-Year-Old Man Who Eats 25 Eggs a Day." *NEJM* 324.13 (28 Mar. 1991): 896–99.

Peplow, P. V. "Modification to Dietary Intake of Sodium, Potassium, Calcium, Magnesium and Trace Elements Can Influence Arachidonic Acid Metabolism and Eicosanoid Production." *Prostaglandins Leukotrienes and Essential Fatty Acids* 45 (1992): 1–19.

Pitt, Bertram, et al. "Design and Recruitment in the United States of a Multicenter Quantitative Angiographic Trial of Pravastatin to Limit Atherosclerosis in the Coronary Arteries (PLAC I)." *American Journal of Cardiology* 72 (1 July 1993): 31–35.

Chapter 6

Ascherio, Alberto, et al. "Dietary Intake of Marine N-3 Fatty Acids, Fish Intake, and the Risk of Coronary Disease Among Men." *NEJM* 332.15 (13 Apr. 1995): 977–82.

Crouce, John Robert, III, et al. "Pravastatin, Lipids, and Atherosclerosis in the Carotid Arteries (PLAC-II)." *American Journal of Cardiology* 75 (1 Mar. 1995): 455–459.

Grundy, Scott M. "Comparison of Monounsaturated Fatty Acids and Carbohydrates for Lowering Plasma Cholesterol." *NEJM* 314.12 (20 Mar. 1986): 745–48.

Levine, Glenn N., et al. "Cholesterol Reduction in Cardiovascular Disease, Clinical Benefits and Possible Mechanisms." *NEJM* 332.8 (23 Feb. 1995): 512–21.

Muldoon, M. F., S. B. Manuck, and K. A. Matthews. "Lowering Cholesterol Concentrations and Mortality: A Quantitative Review of Primary Prevention Trials." *British Medical Journal* 301.6747 (11 Aug. 1990): 309–14.

Reihnér, Eva, et al. "Influence of Pravastatin, a Specific Inhibitor of HMG-CoA Reductase, on Hepatic Metabolism of Cholesterol." *NEJM* 323.4 (26 July 1990): 224–28.

Weintraub, William S., et al. "Lack of Effect of Lovastatin on Re-stenosis After Coronary Angioplasty." *NEJM* 331.20 (17 Nov. 1994): 1331–37.

Chapter 7

Bersohn, A. and I. Antonis. "The Influence of Diet on Serum Triglycerides in South African White and Bantu Prisoners." *Lancet* I.7167 (7 Jan. 1961): 3–9.

Cruz, A. B., D. S. Armatuzzio, F. Grande and L. J. Haye. "Effect of Intraarterial Insulin on Tissue Cholesterol and Fatty Acids in Alloxan-Diabetic Dogs." *Circulation Research.* (1961): 9.39–43.

Ginsburg, H. and S. M. Grundy. "Very Low Density Lipoprotein Metabolism in Non-Ketotic Diabetes Mellitus: Effect of Dietary Restriction." *Diabetologia* 23 (1982): 421–25.

Hjermann, I., et al. "Effect of Diet and Smoking Intervention on the Incidence of Coronary Artery Disease." *Lancet* (12 Dec. 1981): 1303–10.

Keys, Ancel, ed. "Coronary Heart Disease in Seven Countries." *Circulation* 41 supp. #1 (April 1970): I–1–I–211.

Woodard, David A. and Marian C. Limacher. "The Impact of Diet on Coronary Artery Disease." *Clinical Nutrition* 77.4 (July 1993): 849–62.

Chapter 8

Gordon, David J. and Basil M. Rifkind. "Current Concepts-High-Density Lipoprotein—The Clinical Implications of Recent Studies." *NEJM* 321.19 (9 Nov. 1989): 1311–15.

Mensink, Ronald P. and Martijn B. Katan. "Effect of Dietary Transfatty Acids on High-Density and Low-Density Lipoprotein Cholesterol Levels in Healthy Subjects." *NEJM* 323.7 (16 Aug.1990): 439–44.

Reaven, Peter D. and Joseph L. Witztum. "Lipids and Metabolic Disease: The Role of Oxidation of LDL in Atherogenesis." *Endocrinologist* 5.1 (Jan. 1995): 44–52.

Regnstrîm, Jan, et al. "Susceptibility to Low Density Lipoprotein Oxidation and Coronary Atherosclerosis in Men." *Lancet* 339.8803 (16 May 1992): 1183–86.

Steinberg, Daniel, et al. "Beyond Cholesterol: Modifications of Low-Density Lipoprotein That Increase Its Atherogenicity." *NEJM* 320.14 (6 April 1989): 915–23.

Chapter 9

American Heart Association National Center. "Estimated In-patient Cardiovascular Operation, Procedure and Patient Data US 1979–93." Dallas: American Heart Association Office of Scientific Affairs, 1995.

———. "Total Population-Death Rates for Coronary Heart Disease (410–414), by Age, Per 100,000 US, 1979–92." Dallas: American Heart Association Office of Scientific Affairs, 1995.

Bagatell, Carrie J., et al. "Physiologic Testosterone Levels in Normal Men Suppress High-Density Lipoprotein Cholesterol Levels." *Annals of Internal Medicine* 116 (15 June 1992): 967–73.

Colditz, G. A., J. E. Manson, and S. E. Hankinson. "The Nurses' Health Study:

20-Year Contribution to the Understanding of Health Among Women." *Journal of Women's Health* 6.1 (1997): 49–62.

Council on Epidemiology of the American Heart Association and the National Heart, Lung, and Blood Institute. Abstracts of the 31st Annual Conference on Cardiovascular Disease in Orlando, Florida. Vol. 83. No. 2. March 1991.

———. Abstracts of the 34th Annual Conference on Cardiovascular Disease in Tampa, Florida. Vol. 89. No. 2. March 1994.

Després, Jean-Pierre, et al. "Hyperinsulinemia as an Independent Risk Factor For Ischemic Heart Disease." *NEJM* 334.15 (1996 Apr. 11): 952–56.

Hermanson, Bonnie, et al. "Beneficial Six-Year Outcome of Smoking Cessation in Older Men and Women With Coronary Artery Disease: Results from the CASS Registry." *NEJM* 319.21 (24 Nov.1988): 1365–68.

Lipid Research Clinics Program. "The Lipid Research Clinics Coronary Primary Prevention Trial Results to Their Relationship of Reduction in Incidents of Coronary Heart Disease to Cholesterol Lowering." *JAMA* 251.3 (20 Jan.1984.): 365–74.

Manson, JoAnn E., et al. "Prospective Study of Obesity and Risk of Coronary Heart Disease in Women." *NEJM* 322.13 (29 Mar. 1990): 882–89.

Matthews, Karen A., et al. "Menopause and Risk Factors for Coronary Heart Disease." *NEJM* 321.10 (7 Sept. 1989): 641–46.

McGovern, Paul.G., et al. "Recent Trends in Acute Coronary Heart Disease." *NEJM* 334.14 (4 Apr. 1996): 884–89.

Morrow, J. D., et al. "Increase in Circulating Products of Lipid Peroxidation and Smokers: Smoking Is a Cause of Oxidative Damage." *NEJM* 332.18 (4 May 1995): 1198–1203.

Ross, R. "Medical Progress: The Pathogenesis of Atherosclerosis: An Update." *NEJM* 314.8 (20 Feb 1986): 488–500.

Sytkowski, Pamela A., William B. Kannel, and Ralph B. D'Agostino. "Changes in Risk Factors and the Decline in Mortality from Cardiovascular Disease: The Framingham Heart Study." *NEJM* 322.23 (7 June 1990): 1635–40.

Wissler, R. W. "Update on the Pathogenesis of Atherosclerosis." *American Journal of Medicine* 91.1B (31 July 1991): 3S–9S.

Chapter 10

Benowitz, Neal L. "Drug Therapy: Pharmacologic Aspects of Cigarette Smoking and Nicotine Addiction." *NEJM* 319 (17 Nov. 1998): 1318–29.

Brown, W. Virgil. "Lipoprotein Disorders in Diabetes Mellitus." *Medical Clinics of North America* 78.1 (Jan. 1994): 143–61.

Dean, J. D., et al. "Hyperinsulinemia and Microvascular Angina." *Lancet* 337.8739 (23 Feb. 1991): 456–57.

Facchini, F. S., et al. "Insulin Resistance and Cigarette Smoking." *Lancet* 339.8802 (9 May 1992): 1128–30.

Saad, Mohammed F., et al. "Natural History of Impaired Glucose Tolerance in the Pima Indians." *NEJM* 319.23 (8 Dec. 1988): 1500–06.

Chapter 11

Ames, Bruce N., Lois Swirsky Gold, and Walter C. Willett. "The Causes and Prevention of Cancer," *Proc. Natl. Acad. Sci. USA* 92 (1995).

Ayre, Steven G., Donato Perez Garcia y Bellon, and Donato Perez Garcia, Jr. "Insulin Plus Low-Dose CMF as Neo-Adjuvant Chemohormonal Therapy for Breast Carcinoma." Paper presented at the Third International Congress on Neo-Adjuvant Chemotherapy, Paris, Feb. 1992.

Davis, D. L., G. E. Dinse, and D. G. Hoel. "Decreasing Cardiovascular Disease and Increasing Cancer Among Whites in the United States from 1973-1987." *JAMA* 271.6 (9 Feb. 1994): 431–37.

Newman, Thomas B., M.D., M.P.H.; and Stephen B. Hulley, M.D., M.P.H. "Carcinogenicity of Lipid-Lowering Drugs." *The Journal of the American Medical Association*, a Special Communication article. 275.1. (3 Jan. 1996): 55–60.

LeRoith, Derek, et al. "Insulin-like Growth Factors and Cancer." *Annals of Internal Medicine* 122.1 (1 Jan. 1995): 54–59.

Ries, Lynn A. Gloeckler, et al., eds. *Seer Cancer Statistics Review*, 1973-1991: Tables and Graphs. NIH Pub. # 94–2789. Bethesda, Md.: National Cancer Institute, 1994.

Serdula, Mary K., et al. "Weight Control Practices of U.S. Adolescents and Adults." *Annals of Internal Medicine* 19.7 (1 Oct. 1993): 667–71.

Chapter 12

Coulston, Ann M., et al. "Effects of Source of Dietary Carbohydrate on Plasma Glucose and Insulin Responses to Mixed Meals in Subjects with NIDDM." *Diabetes Care* 10.4 (July-Aug. 1987): 395–400.

Jenkins, David J. A., Thomas M. S. Wolever, and Alexandra L. Jenkins. "Starchy Foods and Glycemic Index." *Diabetes Care* 11.2 (Feb. 1988): 149–59.

Chapter 13

Williamson, David F. "Descriptive Epidemiology of Body Weight and Weight Change." *Annals of Internal Medicine* 119.7 (1 Oct. 1993): 646–49.

Chapter 14

See General Overview.

Chapter 15

Coulston, Ann M., et al. "Persistence of Hypertriglyceridemic Effect of Low-Fat, High-Carbohydrate Diets In NIDDM Patients." *Diabetes Care* 12.2 (Feb. 1989): 94–101.

Garg, Abhimanyu, et al. "Comparison of a High-Carbohydrate Diet with a High-Monounsaturated-Fat Diet in Patients with Non-Insulin-Dependent Diabetes Mellitus." *NEJM* 319.13 (29 Sept. 1988): 829–34.

National Institutes of Health. "Consensus Development Conference on Diet and Exercise in Non-Insulin-Dependent Diabetes Mellitus." *Diabetes Care* 10.5 (Sept./Oct. 1987): 639–44.

Chapter 16

Horm, John and Kay Anderson. "Who in America Is Trying to Lose Weight?" *Annals of Internal Medicine* 119.7 (1 Oct. 1993): 672–76.

Hyman, Frederick N., et al. "Evidence for Success of Calorie Restriction in Weight Loss and Control." *Annals of Internal Medicine* 119.7 (1 Oct. 1993): 681–87.

Leiter, Lawrence, et al. "Obesity and Dyslipidemia: Epidemiology, Physiology, and Effects of Weight Loss." *Endocrinologist* 5.2 (Mar. 1995): 118–131.

Levy, Alan S. and Alan W. Heaton. "Weight Control Practices of U. S. Adults Trying to Lose Weight." *Annals of Internal Medicine* 119.7 (part 2) (1 Oct. 1993): 661–666.

Nestler, John E. and Daniela J. Jakubowicz. "Decreases in Ovarian

Cytochrome P450c17∝ Activity and Serum Free Testosterone after Reduction of Insulin Secretion in Polycystic Ovary Syndrome." *NEJM* 335.9 (29 Aug. 1996): 617–623.

Peiris, A. N., et al. "Relative Contributions of Hepatic and Peripheral Tissues to Insulin Resistance in Hyperandrogenic Women." *Journal of Clinical Endocrinology & Metabolism* 68.4 (Apr. 1989): 715–20.

Rodin, Judith. "Cultural Psychosocial Determinants of Weight Concerns." *Annals of Internal Medicine* 119.7 (1 Oct. 1993): 643–45.

Wild, Robert A. "Metabolic and Cardiovascular Issues in Women with Androgen Excess." *Endocrinologist* 6.2 (Mar. 1996): 120–124.

Chapter 17

See General Overview.

Chapter 18

Steinberg, K. K., et al. "Sex Steroids and Bone Density in Premenopausal and Perimenopausal Women." *Journal of Clinical Endocrinology & Metabolism* 69.3 (Sept. 1989): 533–39.

Wilson, Jean D., et al., eds. *Williams Textbook of Endocrinology.* 9th ed. Philadelphia: W. B. Saunders, 1998.

Chapter 26

Matthews, Ruth H., Pamela R. Pehrsson, and Moigan Farhat-Sabet. Sugar Content of Selected Foods: Individual and Total Sugars. Home Economics

Research Report #48. Riverdale, Md.: USDA Human Nutrition Information Service, 1987.

Chapter 27

Kinsella, J. E., et al. "Metabolism of *Trans* Fatty Acids with Emphasis on the Effects of *Trans, Trans*-octadecadienoate on Lipid Composition, Essential Fatty Acid, and Prostaglandins: An Overview." *The American Journal of Clinical Nutrition* 34 (Oct. 1981): 2307–18.

Pennington, J. T. *Bowes & Church's Food Values of Portions Commonly Used.* 16th ed. Philadelphia: J. B. Lippincott, 1994.

Steinman, David. *Diet for a Poisoned Planet: How to Choose Safe Foods for You and Your Family.* New York: Ballantine Books, 1990.

Thomas, Leo H. "Mortality from Arteriosclerotic Disease and Consumption of Hydrogenated Oils and Fats." *Britt. J. prev. soc. Med* 29 (1975): 82–90.

Thomas, Leo H., et al. "Hydrogenated Oils and Fats: The Presence of Chemically Modified Fatty Acids in Human Adipose Tissue." *The American Journal of Clinical Nutrition* 34 (May 1981): 877–86.

Winter, Ruth. *A Consumer's Dictionary of Food Additives.* New York: Crown Trade Paperbacks, 1994.

Index

A

accelerated metabolic aging, 3–16
  alcohol's role in, 12, 285
  from carbohydrates, 8, 10–11
  cellular aging, 4–5
  committed cells, 4–5
  defined, xxiv, 5–6
  degenerative diseases, acquired,
    12–16
  factors accelerating, 6
  fat's role in, 11
  healing program for, 10–11
  hormones and aging, 4, 5, 13
  hyperinsulinemia, 8
  "insulin meter," 10, 100
  insulin resistance, 6–12, 16
  insulin's role in, 6–14, 15, 16
  metabolism, defined, 3–4, 5
  protein's role in, 12
  quiz, 224–25
  from smoking, 103–7
  stem cells, 4–5
  water's role in, 12
acne, 168
activity level and carbohydrates needed,
  259–60
ADD (attention deficit disorder), 52
addictions, 42–43.
  See also sugar addiction

age
  and cancer, 110, 112
  and heart disease, 98
aging. See accelerated metabolic aging;
  food chain; hormones and fat; low-
  serotonin state
alcohol, avoiding, 12, 285
American Diabetes Association (ADA),
  xvi, xvii, xviii
American restaurants tips, 337
amino acids and hormones, 24
anorexia nervosa, 177
antidepressants, 48–50
Anytime Soup, 331
aspartame, avoiding, 285
asthma, 168–69
atherosclerosis (plaqueing of arteries),
  81–82, 94–97, 102
attention deficit disorder (ADD), 52

B

balanced diet, 35–36, 123–24.
  See also Healing Program; low-fat
  diet dangers; Maintenance Program;
  Schwarzbein Principle
Beef Stroganoff, Classic, 333
body
  composition, ideal, 228–30
  interconnected, 209–14

body fat
  defined, 63
  gaining, 133–40
  loss and diet scams, 154–58
bone formation, 179–83
brain function, 21, 23
bread, 269
Broccoli Cheese Pie, 332
bulimia, 177

C
caffeine, avoiding, 285
calcium, 46, 272
calorie
  defined, 127–29
  restricted diets, 154–58
  See also low-fat diet dangers
cancer, 109–16
  and age, 110, 112
  from carbohydrates, 113–14
  from cholesterol-lowering drugs, 113
  from fats, damaged, 113
  fat's role in, 110, 113, 115
  and genetics, 114
  and hormones, 110–11, 113, 114–15
  and immune system, 112–13, 115
  and insulin, 109–16
  risk factors, 110–12
  from stimulants, 114
  from stress, 115
  from toxin exposure, 114
carbohydrates as sugar, 119–26
  accelerated metabolic aging, 8, 10–11
  balanced meals, 35–36, 123–24
  cholecystokinin (CCK), 124
  complex carbohydrates, 119
  with fats, 121, 123, 124
  and glucagon, 119–23, 124
  glycemic index of foods, 122, 123
  healing program for, 126
  insulin-to-glucagon ratio,
    119–23, 124
  overeating, 124–26, 138
  with proteins, 121, 123, 124

serotonin, 126
simple carbohydrates, 119
stored as fat, 121, 123
  See also carbohydrates nutrient
    group; carbohydrates' role
carbohydrates nutrient group, 259–71
  activity level and amount needed,
    259–60
  bread, 269
  consumption guidelines, 259–60
  crackers, 270
  fruits, 266–68
  grains, 263
  juices, 270–71
  legumes, 262
  liquid, 270–71
  man-made, 269–70
  overeating, 124–26, 138
  starchy vegetables, 261
  tips for, 271
  whole-grain flour/meals, 264
  yogurt, 265
  See also carbohydrates as sugar;
    carbohydrates' role; nonstarchy
    vegetables nutrient group
carbohydrates' role
  in cancer, 113–14
  "carbo-loading" dangers, 137, 139
  cholesterol and fat from, 68–71
  in cravings, 170–71, 207–8
  in food chain, 36–37
  overeating, 124–26, 138
  in proteins, 247–48
  in Schwarzbein Principle, xvii–xx,
    xxiii, xxiv
  as stimulants, 42, 43, 48, 178–79
  in vegetarian diet, 205, 207–8
  See also carbohydrates as sugar;
    carbohydrates nutrient group
"carbo-loading" dangers, 137, 139
carnitine, 272–73
CCK (cholecystokinin), 124
cellular aging, 4–5
cellulite, 185–87

changing lifestyle, 217–20
cheese, 246
Cheese Broccoli Pie, 332
chemical ingestion, 29, 31, 114
Chicken Frittata, Spicy, 326
Chicken Salad, Chinese, 327
children, overweight, 195–99
    adrenarche, puberty, 196
    low-fat, high carbohydrate diet
    dangers, 196–97
Chinese Chicken Salad, 327
Chinese restaurants tips, 337
cholecystokinin (CCK), 124
cholesterol and fat, 61–71
    body fat, 63, 133–40, 154–58
    from carbohydrates, 68–71
    cholesterol, functions of, 62–63
    dietary fats, 63, 70
    eicosanoids, 64–65
    essential fatty acids, 64–65
    fat storage, insulin for, 63, 152–53,
    159
    fats, functions of, 63–64
    HMG Co-A Reductase enzyme,
    69, 70
    insulin's role in, 63, 69, 70, 71
    linoleic acid, 64–65
    linolenic acid, 64–65
    liver's role in, 67–68, 69
    for regeneration, 61, 64
    structural fats, 63
    See also cholesterol count
cholesterol count, 75–84
    cholesterol-lowering drugs, cancer
    from, 113
    fat's role in, 86
    and heart disease, 76, 78, 79–80, 86
    high-density lipoproteins (HDLs),
    75–76, 85–91, 90
    insulin's role in, 81–84
    lipoproteins, 75–78
    low-density lipoproteins (LDLs),
    75–76, 89, 90
    numbers, focus on, 79–81, 82–83, 88

plaqueing of arteries
    (atherosclerosis), 81–82, 94–97,
    102
    protein's role in, 87
    smoking, impact on, 80
    triglycerides, 75–76
    very low-density lipoproteins
    (VLDLs), 75–76, 89, 90
    See also cholesterol and fat;
    heart disease
chromium, 273
Classic Beef Stroganoff, 333
claudication from smoking, 105
committed cells, 4–5
complex carbohydrates, 119
condiments, avoiding, 284
cooking with fats, 279, 281
corn syrup, avoiding, 285, 286
cortisol levels, 186–86
Cottage Cheese Salad with Chopped
    Vegetables, 328
crackers, 270
cravings
    from low-serotonin state, 42–43
    and sugar addiction, 170–71
    and vegetarian diet, 207–8
cyanocobalamin (B₁₂), 273
Cytomel, 49

D
degenerative diseases, acquired,
    xxi–xxii, 12–16
delayed puberty, 167–68
desserts, avoiding, 283
Dexedrine, 49
dextrose, avoiding, 286
diabetes
    experiences with, xvi–xxiii
    Type II diabetes, 101–2
Diabetes Care, 82
diet scams, 149–62
    body fat loss, 63, 133–40, 154–58
    calorie-restricted diets, 154–58
    diet industry victims, 150–52

diet scams *(continued)*
    fat-storage system, insulin directed,
        63, 152–53, 159
    infertility and stress, 158–62
    insulin directed, fat-storage system,
        63, 152–53, 159
    insulin levels and Stein-Leventhal
        Syndrome (SLS), 157–58
    muscle mass, losing, 135–36, 155
    prehistoric humans, 17, 152–53
    Stein-Leventhal Syndrome (SLS),
        157–58
    stress and infertility, 158–62
    yo-yo dieting, 155–56
    See also children, overweight; fats do
        not make you fat; low-fat diet
        dangers; overfed and undernour-
        ished; sugar addiction; thin, being
        too
dietary fats, 63, 70
dining out tips, 336–40
drugs, elimination of, 236–37

E
eating disorders. *See* children, over-
    weight; diet scams; fats do not make
    you fat; low-fat diet dangers; overfed
    and undernourished; sugar addiction;
    thin, being too
"Effect of Diet and Smoking Intervention
    on the Incidence of Coronary Heart
    Disease," 79–80
Eggplant Parmigiana, 334
eggs
    as protein, 244
    in vegetarian diet, 205, 206
eicosanoids, 64–65, 169
energy and calories, 127–29
essential fatty acids
    for human life, 64–65
    for serotonin, 46
    as supplements, 272
estrogen
    for serotonin, 44–45

and sugar addiction, 170–71
exercise
    bone damage from, 182
    and heart disease, 90–91
    in Schwarzbein Principle, 233–35

F
fast foods, avoiding, 286–88
fats, damaged, 277–88
    avoiding, guidelines, 281
    cancer from, 113
    cooking with, 279, 281
    hydrogenated fats as, 280
    monounsaturated fats, 279
    from oxidation, 280
    polyunsaturated oils, 278–79
    saturated fats, 279
    tips for, 281–82
    trans-fatty acids as, 278–79
    See also fats do not make you fat;
        fats nutrient group; fat's role;
        free radicals
fats do not make you fat, 127–32
    calories, defined, 127–29
    energy and calories, 127–29
    low-fat, high-carbohydrate diet,
        dangers, 129–32
    See also fats, damaged; fats nutrient
        group; fat's role
fats nutrient group, 251–55
    monounsaturated fats, 251–52,
        254, 279
    oils, best to use, 254
    overeating, 124–25, 251
    polyunsaturated fats, 252, 254,
        278–79
    "pure-pressed oils," 253, 254
    saturated fats, 251, 252, 253, 254,
        279
    tips for, 255
    See also fats, damaged; fats do not
        make you fat; fat's role
fat's role
    in accelerated metabolic aging, 11

in cancer, 110, 113, 115
with carbohydrates, 121, 123, 124
in cholesterol count, 86
functions of, 63–64
and hormones, 20, 22, 27
overeating, 124–25, 251
in Schwarzbein Principle, xix, xxi,
    xxiii, xxiv
See also cholesterol and fat; fats,
    damaged; fats do not make you
    fat; fats nutrient group; hor-
    mones and fat
fat-storage system, insulin directed, 63,
    152–53, 159
feedback mechanisms
    for carbohydrates overeating,
        124–26, 138
    for fats overeating, 124–25, 251
    for proteins overeating, 124–25, 244
"fight-or-flight," 101
Fish, Greek-Style Baked, 335
fish and shellfish, 246
5-hydroxytryptophan (5-HTP), 46, 272
folate, 273
food chain, 29–38
    balanced nutrition, 35–36, 123–24
    carbohydrates' role in, 36–37
    and chemical ingestion, 29, 31, 114
    defined, 30, 32
    "food products," 29, 33, 36, 37
    food pyramid, USDA, 34
    free radicals, 32–33
    hormone balance and nutrient
        groups, 35
    Industrial Revolution impact on,
        29, 31
    insulin and stimulants, 36
    ketones, 37
    nutrient groups, 34–38, 244–75
    regeneration process, 30, 35
    Schwarzbein Square (nutrient
        groups), 34–38, 244–75
    stimulants, 36

"food products," avoiding, 29, 33, 36,
    37, 269–70, 282–84
food pyramid, USDA, 34
foods to avoid
    alcohol, 12, 285
    aspartame, 285
    caffeine, 285
    condiments, 284
    corn syrup, 285, 286
    desserts, 283
    dextrose, 286
    fast foods, 286–88
    fructose, 285, 286
    grain products, refined, 283
    maltodextrin, 286
    maltose, 286
    man-made products, 29, 33, 36, 37,
        269–70, 282–84
    molasses, 286
    Olestra (Olean), 195, 285
    polydextrose, 286
    processed foods, 282, 284, 285–86
    refined foods, 283, 285–86
    saccharin, 286
    salt, 286
    sausages, processed, 282
    snack foods, processed, 284
    sorbital, 286
    sucrose, 286
    sugar, 283
    tobacco, 286
    See also fats, damaged
free radicals, 32–33
French restaurants tips, 337
Frittata, Spicy Chicken, 326
fructose, avoiding, 285, 286
fruits, 266–68

G
gamma-linolenic acid, 46
gender and heart disease, 98
genetics
    and cancer, 114
    and heart disease, 98–99

glucagon, 119–23, 124
gluten sensitivity, 169–70
glycemic index of foods, 122, 123
glycogen, 21, 22
grains, 263
grains, refined, avoiding, 283
Greek-Style Baked Fish, 335

H
hair damage, 185–87
HDLs (high-density lipoproteins),
 75–76, 85–91, 90
headaches and serotonin, 193
Healing Program
 for carbohydrates excess, 126
 defined, 10–11, 241–42
 for hormones, 24–26
 meal planning for, 292–306
 vegetarian, meal planning for,
 308–22
 See also carbohydrates nutrient
 group; fats, damaged; fats nutrient group; foods to avoid; meal
 planning; nonstarchy vegetables
 nutrient group; protein nutrient
 group; vitamins and minerals
heart disease
 and age, 98
 cholesterol count, 76, 78, 79–80, 86
 from cholesterol metabolism,
 abnormal, 98
 and exercise, 90–91
 and gender, 98
 and genetics, 98–99
 from high blood pressure, 99
 and hormone replacement therapy,
 100
 from insulin levels, high, xxi, xxiii,
 99–100
 from "insulin meter," 10, 100
 and low-fat diets, 90–91
 and menopausal status, 100
 from plaqueing of arteries (atherosclerosis), 81–82, 94–97, 102

risk factors, 93–102
 from sedentary lifestyle, 100–101
 from smoking, 101
 from stimulants, 101
 from stress, 101
 and Type II diabetes, 101–2
 See also cholesterol and fat;
 cholesterol count
high blood pressure, 99
high-carbohydrate, low-fat diet,
 129–32. See also low-fat diet dangers
high-density lipoproteins (HDLs),
 75–76, 85–91, 90
high-insulin
 and cancer, 109–16
 habits quiz, 225–26
 lowering, 226–27
 See also insulin
HMG Co-A Reductase, 69, 70
hormone replacement therapy
 and heart disease, 100
 in Schwarzbein Principle, 237–38
 for serotonin, 45, 46
hormones
 and aging, 4, 5, 13
 balance and nutrient groups, 35
 and cancer, 110–11, 113, 114–15
 See also hormone replacement
 therapy; hormones and fat
hormones and fat, 17–27
 amino acids' role in, 24
 for brain function, 21, 23
 fat's role in, 20, 22, 27
 glycogen, 21, 22
 healing program for, 24–26
 hydrochloric acid, 25
 immune system, 24
 immunoglobulins, 24
 low-fat diets, dangers, 18–24, 26, 27
 malnutrition, 23
 metabolism, 20, 21–24, 26
 prehistoric humans, 17, 152–53
 protein's role in, 20, 22, 24–27
 for regeneration, 20–21, 22, 24

"water weight," 22
See also hormone replacement
    therapy; hormones
hydrochloric acid, 25
hydrogenated fats, 280
hyperinsulinemia, 8
"Hyperinsulinemia as an Independent
    Risk Factor for Ischemic Heart
    Disease," 100
hypoglycemia (low blood sugar),
    178–79
hypothyroidism, 50

I
ideal body composition, 228–30
immune system
    and cancer, 112–13, 115
    hormones and fat for, 24
immunoglobulins, 24
Industrial Revolution impact on food
    chain, 29, 31
infertility and stress, 158–62
insomnia and serotonin, 52–53, 193
"Insulin and Atheroma: Twenty-Year
    Perspective," 82
"insulin meter," 10, 100
insulin resistance
    accelerated metabolic aging from,
        6–12, 16
    defined, xviii, xxii
    from low-serotonin, 55–56
    from smoking, 104–5
    See also high-insulin; insulin's role
insulin's role
    in accelerated metabolic aging,
        6–14, 15, 16
    in cancer, 114
    in cholesterol, 63, 69, 70, 71
    in cholesterol count, 81–84
    in fat-storage, 63, 152–53, 159
    in heart disease, xxi, xxiii, 99–100
    insulin-to-glucagon ratio, 119–23,
        124

in Schwarzbein Principle, xviii–xix,
    xxi–xxiii
in serotonin, 44, 55–56
and Stein-Leventhal Syndrome
    (SLS), 157–58
and stimulants, 36
See also high-insulin; insulin
    resistance
insulin-to-glucagon ratio, 119–23, 124
irritable bowel syndrome, 169–70
Italian restaurants tips, 336

J
Jaffe, Evelyn Jacob, 289
Japanese restaurants tips, 338
journal for programs, 230
juices, 270–71

K
ketones, 37

L
LDLs (low-density lipoproteins), 75–76,
    89, 90
legumes, 262
lifestyle, changing, 217–20
linoleic acid, 64–65
linolenic acid, 64–65
lipoproteins, 75–78
liquid carbohydrates, 270–71
liver's role
    in cholesterol, 67–68, 69
    and insulin, xviii
longevity and serotonin, 53–54
low blood sugar (hypoglycemia),
    178–79
low-density lipoproteins (LDLs), 75–76,
    89, 90
low-fat diet dangers
    beliefs, dispelling, 141–46
    body fat, gaining, 133–40
    calorie, defined, 127–29
    calorie-restricted diets, 154–58
    carbohydrate overeating, signs of,
        124–26, 138

low-fat diet dangers *(continued)*
  "carbo-loading" dangers, 137, 139
  and heart disease, 90–91
  and high-carbohydrate, results of,
    129–32
  and hormones, 18–24, 26, 27
  muscle mass, losing, 135–36, 155
  overview, xix, xx–xxi, xxiii–xxiv
  and serotonin, 54–57
  symptoms of, 137
  See also children, overweight; diet
    scams; fats do not make you fat;
    overfed and undernourished;
    sugar addiction; thin, being too
low-serotonin state, 39–57
  addictions, curing, 42–43
  from antidepressants, 48–50
  attention deficit disorder (ADD)
    from, 52
  carbohydrates as stimulants, 42,
    43, 48
  cravings from, 42–43
  essential fatty acids for, 46
  estrogen for, 44–45
  gamma-linolenic acid for, 46
  hormone replacement therapy for,
    45, 46
  hypothyroidism, 50
  insomnia from, 52–53, 193
  insulin resistance from, 55–56
  insulin's role in, 44, 55–56
  and longevity, 53–54
  low-fat dieting dangers, 54–57
  magnesium for, 45
  melatonin production, 53
  and metabolism, 40–42, 56
  moods affected by, 39–40
  "noise" (demand for stimulants),
    42, 44
  omega-3 and 6 for, 46
  protein's role in, 44
  raising levels naturally, 43–46
  from starvation, 47–48
  from stimulants, 40–43, 47, 48, 55-56
  from stress, 46–47
  supplements for, 46
  and thyroid, 50–52
  tryptophan for, 44, 45
  vitamin B$_6$ for, 45
  See also serotonin
L-tryptophan, 46, 272
lunch meats, 245

M
magnesium, 45, 46, 272, 273
Maintenance Program, 243. *See also*
  carbohydrates nutrient group; fats,
  damaged; fats nutrient group; foods
  to avoid; meal planning; nonstarchy
  vegetables nutrient group; protein
  nutrient group; vitamins and
  minerals
malnutrition, 23, 189–94
maltodextrin, avoiding, 286
maltose, avoiding, 286
man-made food products, avoiding,
  29, 33, 36, 37, 269–70, 282–84
meal planning, 289–321
  in American restaurants, 337
  Anytime Soup, 331
  Broccoli Cheese Pie, 332
  Chinese Chicken Salad, 327
  in Chinese restaurants, 337
  Classic Beef Stroganoff, 333
  Cottage Cheese Salad with Chopped
    Vegetables, 328
  dining out tips, 336–40
  Eggplant Parmigiana, 334
  in French restaurants, 337
  Greek-Style Baked Fish, 335
  for healing program, 292–306
  for healing program, vegetarian,
    308–22
  in Italian restaurants, 336
  in Japanese restaurants, 338
  in Mexican restaurants, 338
  Nancy Deville's Crustless Spinach
    and Mushroom Quiche, 323

Salad Niçoise, 329
San Francisco Joe's Special, 324
Soy Sausage Tofu Scramble, 325
Spicy Chicken Frittata, 326
Tofu "Egg" Salad, 330
for vegetarians, healing program, 308–22
meat, 245
melatonin and serotonin, 53
menopause
and heart disease, 100
and osteoporosis, 182
metabolism
defined, 3–4, 5
hormones and fat for, 20, 21–24, 26
and serotonin, 40–42, 56
stimulants' destruction of, 40–42
methyl-testosterone, 238
Mexican restaurants tips, 338
midsection body-fat gain, 10, 100
minerals. See vitamins and minerals
molasses, avoiding, 286
monounsaturated fats, 251–52, 254, 279
moods and serotonin, 39–40
multivitamins, 46, 272
muscle mass, losing, 135–36, 155
Mushroom and Spinach Quiche, Nancy Deville's Crustless, 323

N
Nancy Deville's Crustless Spinach and Mushroom Quiche, 323
New England Journal of Medicine, The, 99–100
niacin (B₃), 273
Niçoise Salad, 329
"noise" (demand for stimulants), 42, 44, 177–79
nonstarchy vegetables nutrient group, 256–58
condiments, 258
herbs and spices, 258
tips for, 258

"Nurses' Health Study: Twenty-Year Contribution to the Understanding of Health Among Women," 98–99
nutrient groups, 34–38, 244–75
nutrition, 227–30
nuts, nut butters and seeds, 247–48

O
oils, best to use, 254
Olestra (Olean), avoiding, 195, 285
omega-3 and 6, 46
optimum health, 227–28
osteopenia, 181
osteoporosis, 179–85
overeating
carbohydrates, 124–26, 138
fats, 124–25, 251
proteins, 124–25, 244
overfed and undernourished, 189–94
ovo-lacto-vegetarian guidelines, 249–50
oxidation and fats, 280

P
Parmigiana, Eggplant, 334
Pie, Broccoli Cheese, 332
plaqueing of arteries (atherosclerosis), 81–82, 94–97, 102
polydextrose, avoiding, 286
polyunsaturated fats, 252, 254, 278–79
poultry, 245
prehistoric humans, 17, 152–53
Premarin, 238
Pritikin Diet, 19
processed foods, avoiding, 282, 284, 285–86
protein nutrient group, 244–50
carbohydrates in, 247–48
cheese, 246
eggs, 244
fish and shellfish, 246
lunch meats, 245
meat, 245
nuts, nut butters and seeds, 247–48
overeating, 124–25, 244

protein nutrient group *(continued)*
  ovo-lacto-vegetarian guidelines,
    249–50
  poultry, 245
  sausages, 245
  soy products, 248
  tips for, 249
  vegetarian guidelines, 249–50
  See also protein's role
protein's role
  in accelerated metabolic aging, 12
  with carbohydrates, 121, 123, 124
  in cholesterol count, 87
  in hormones and fat, 20, 22, 24–27
  overeating, 124–25, 244
  in Schwarzbein Principle, xix
  in serotonin, 44
  in vegetarian diet, 205
  See also protein nutrient group
Provera, 238
Prozac, 48–49
"pure-pressed oils," 253, 254
pyridoxine (B$_6$), 45, 46, 272, 273–74

Q
Quiche, Nancy Deville's Spinach and
  Mushroom, 323

R
refined foods, avoiding, 283, 285–86
regeneration process
  cholesterol and fat for, 61, 64
  and food chain, 30, 35
  hormones and fat for, 20–21, 22, 24
Respiratory Quotient (RQ), 169
riboflavin (B$_2$), 274

S
saccharin, avoiding, 286
Salad, Chinese Chicken, 327
Salad, Cottage Cheese, with Chopped
  Vegetables, 328
Salad, Tofu "Egg," 330
Salad Niçoise, 329
salt, avoiding, 286

San Francisco Joe's Special, 324
saturated fats, 251, 252, 253, 254, 279
Sausage, Soy, Tofu Scramble, 325
sausages, 245
sausages, avoiding processed, 282
Schwarzbein Principle, 223–39
  defined, xxv
  degenerative diseases, acquired,
    xxi–xxii
  and diabetes experiences, xvi–xxiii
  drugs, elimination, 236–37
  exercise, 233–35
  high-insulin, 225–27
  hormone replacement therapy,
    237–38
  for ideal body composition, 228–30
  journal for, 230
  liver's role in, xviii
  nutrition, 227–30
  for optimum health, 227–28
  researching, xv–xxvii
  stimulants, elimination of, 236–37
  stress management, 230–33
  time to heal, 238–39
  See also accelerated metabolic aging;
    carbohydrates; fats; foods to
    avoid; Healing Program; heart
    disease; insulin; low-fat diet dan-
    gers; Maintenance Program; meal
    planning; nonstarchy vegetables;
    protein; vitamin and minerals
Schwarzbein Principle Cookbook, The
  (Jaffe), 289, 292
*Schwarzbein Principle Vegetarian
  Cookbook, The* (Jaffe), 289, 292
Schwarzbein Square (nutrient groups),
  34–38, 244–75
sedentary lifestyle and heart disease,
  100–101
senile osteoporosis, 182
serotonin
  being too thin, impact on, 178
  and carbohydrates, 126
  and headaches, 193

and insomnia, 52–53, 193
See also low-serotonin state
simple carbohydrates, 119
SLS (Stein-Leventhal Syndrome), 157–58
smoking
  accelerated metabolic aging from, 103–7
  avoiding, 286
  cholesterol, impact on, 80
  claudication from, 105
  heart disease from, 101
  insulin resistance from, 104–5
snack foods, avoiding processed, 284
sorbital, avoiding, 286
Soup, Anytime, 331
soy products, 248
Soy Sausage Tofu Scramble, 325
Spicy Chicken Frittata, 326
Spinach and Mushroom Quiche, Nancy Deville's Crustless, 323
St. John's wort, 46, 50, 272
starchy vegetables, 261
starvation, 47–48, 173–77
Statin drugs, 70–71
Stein-Leventhal Syndrome (SLS), 157–58
stem cells, 4–5
stimulants
  cancer from, 114
  carbohydrates as, 178–79
  elimination of, 236–37
  and food chain, 36
  heart disease from, 101
  low-serotonin from, 40–43, 47, 48, 55–56
  "noise" (demand for), 42, 44, 177–79
stress
  cancer from, 115
  heart disease from, 101
  infertility from, 158–62
  low-serotonin from, 46–47
  management, 230–33
Stroganoff, Classic Beef, 333

structural fats, 63
sucrose, avoiding, 286
sugar, avoiding, 283
sugar addiction, 163–72
  acne from, 168
  asthma from, 168–69
  and carbohydrate craving, 170–71
  delayed puberty from, 167–68
  as eating disorder, 171–72
  and eicosanoids, 169
  and estrogen, low, 170–71
  gluten sensitivity, 169–70
  irritable bowel syndrome, 169–70
  Respiratory Quotient (RQ), 169
supplements, 46, 50, 272.
  See also vitamins and minerals

T
testosterone levels, 185–86
thiamine (B_1), 274
thin, being too, 173–87
  anorexia nervosa, 177
  bone formation, 179–83
  bulimia, 177
  carbohydrates as stimulants, 178–79
  cellulite from, 185–87
  cortisol levels, 185–86
  exercise and bone damage, 182
  hair damage from, 185–87
  hypoglycemia (low blood sugar), 178–79
  menopausal osteoporosis, 182
  "noise" (demand for stimulants), 177–79
  osteopenia from, 181
  osteoporosis from, 179–85
  senile osteoporosis, 182
  serotonin levels, 178
  starving yourself, 173–77
  stimulants, carbohydrates as, 178–79
  testosterone levels, 185–86
  wrinkles from, 186–87
thyroid and serotonin, 50–52
time to heal, 238–39

tobacco. *See* smoking
Tofu "Egg" Salad, 330
Tofu Soy Sausage Scramble, 325
toxin exposure, 29, 31, 114
trans-fatty acids, 278–79
triglycerides, 75–76
tryptophan, 44, 45
Type II diabetes
   experiences with, xvi–xxiii
   and heart disease, 101–2

U
undernourished and overfed, 189–94

V
Vegetables, Chopped, with Cottage
   Cheese Salad, 328
vegetarian diet, 203–14
   body is interconnected, 209–14
   carbohydrate craving, 207–8
   and carbohydrates, 205, 207–8
   and eggs, 205, 206
   guidelines for, 249–50
   healing program for, 308–22
   protein for, 205
very low-density lipoproteins (VLDLs),
   75–76, 89, 90
vitamin A, 274
vitamin B_1 (thiamine), 274
vitamin B_2 (riboflavin), 274
vitamin B_3 (niacin), 273
vitamin B_6 (pyridoxine), 45, 46, 272,
   273–74
vitamin B_{12} (cyanocobalamin), 273

vitamin C, 274
vitamin E, 274
vitamins and minerals, 272–75
   calcium, 272
   carnitine, 272–73
   chromium, 273
   cyanocobalamin (B_{12}), 273
   folate, 273
   magnesium, 273
   multi-vitamins, 46, 272
   niacin (B_3), 273
   pyridoxine (B_6), 45, 46, 272, 273–74
   riboflavin (B_2), 274
   supplements, 46, 50, 272
   thiamine (B_1), 274
   tips for, 275
   vitamin A, 274
   vitamin C, 274
   vitamin E, 274
VLDLs (very low-density lipoproteins),
   75–76, 89, 90

W
water, drinking, 12, 270
"water weight," 22
whole-grain flour/meals, 264
wrinkles, 186–87

Y
yogurt, 265
yo-yo dieting, 155–56

Z
Zoloft, 48–49

About the Authors

Diana Schwarzbein, M.D., graduated from the University of Southern California (USC) Medical School and completed her residency in internal medicine and a fellowship in endocrinology at Los Angeles County USC Medical Center. She founded The Endocrinology Institute of Santa Barbara in 1993. She sub-specializes in metabolism, diabetes, osteoporosis, menopause and thyroid conditions, subjects she lectures on frequently. She lives with her husband in Santa Barbara, California.

Nancy Deville is a writer of nonfiction and fiction with a talent for making science easy to read and understand. She recently completed a novel and screenplay about trafficking in women. She is currently at work on a second novel and nonfiction book. She is a contributing writer on *Legacy: Secrets of Family Business Dynasties*, to be published by St. Martin's Press. She lives with her husband in Santa Barbara, California.

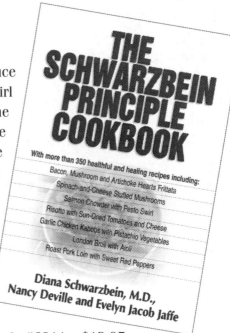

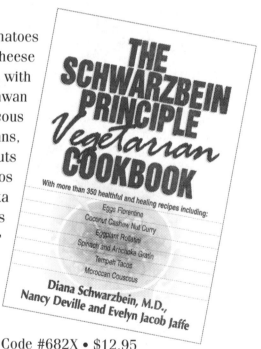

New Chicken Soup for the Soul

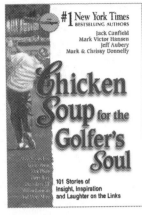

Chicken Soup for the Golfer's Soul

This inspiring collection of stories from professionals, caddies and amateur golfers shares the memorable moments of the game—when, despite all odds, an impossible shot lands in the perfect position; when a simple game of golf becomes a lesson in life. Chapters include: sportsmanship, family, overcoming obstacles, perfecting the game and the nineteenth hole. This is a great read for any golfer, no matter what their handicap.

Code #6587 • $12.95

A 6th Bowl of Chicken Soup for the Soul

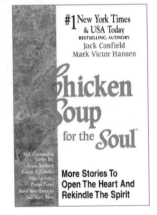

This latest batch of wisdom, love and inspiration will warm your hearts and nourish your souls, whether you're "tasting" *Chicken Soup* for the first time, or have dipped your "spoon" many times before.

In the tradition of all the books in the original *Chicken Soup* series, this volume focuses on love; parents and parenting; teaching and learning; death and dying; perspective; overcoming obstacles; and eclectic wisdom. Contributors to *A 6th Bowl of Chicken Soup for the Soul* include: Erma Bombeck, Edgar Guest, Jay Leno, Rachel Naomi Remen, Robert A. Schuller, Dr. James Dobson, Dolly Parton and Cathy Rigby.

Code #6625 • $12.95

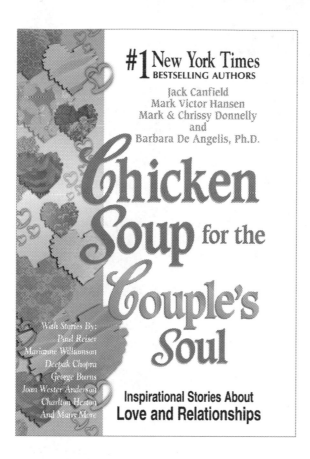

More from the *Chicken Soup for the Soul*® Series

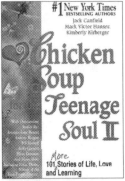

#6161—$12.95

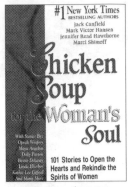

#4150—$12.95

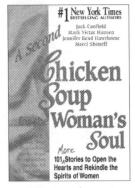

#6218—$12.95

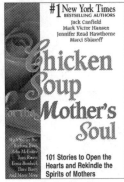

#4606—$12.95

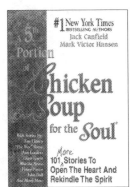

Chicken Soup for the Soul® Series

Each one of these inspiring *New York Times* bestsellers brings you exceptional stories, tales and verses guaranteed to lift your spirits, soothe your soul and warm your heart! A perfect gift for anyone you love, including yourself!

A 5th Portion of Chicken Soup for the Soul, #5432—$12.95
A 4th Course of Chicken Soup for the Soul, #4592—$12.95
A 3rd Serving of Chicken Soup for the Soul, #3790—$12.95
A 2nd Helping of Chicken Soup for the Soul, #3316—$12.95
Chicken Soup for the Soul, #262X—$12.95

Selected books are also available in hardcover, large print, audiocassette and compact disc.

Available in bookstores everywhere or call **1-800-441-5569** for Visa or MasterCard orders. Prices do not include shipping and handling. Your response code is **BKS**. Order online at *www.hci-online.com*.

HCI's Spring Spirituality Series

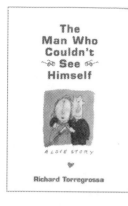

The Man Who Couldn't See Himself

Whimsically illustrated, this is the story of a man who has lost sight of who he is. Filled with loneliness he buys himself a dog, but before long, they are both lonely. Thus begins a sublime journey of a man to rediscover himself. In time and almost imperceptibly he realizes a shift in consciousness and becomes open to the mystery of love.

Code #6781 • $7.95

Ignite Your Intuition

Extraordinist Craig Karges is known to millions of television viewers for his remarkable demonstrations of extraordinary phenomena on *The Tonight Show with Jay Leno, Larry King Live*, and many other TV shows. In his new book, Karges reveals how to unlock the power within your own intuition—what he calls your natural psychic abilities. Be awakened to the possibility of realizing your own potential.

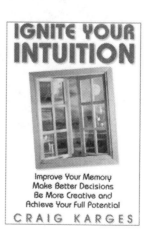

Code # 6765 • $10.95

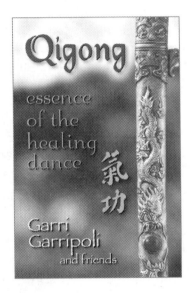